OVERCOME your SEDENTARY LIFESTYLE

(A Practical Guide to Improving Health, Fitness, and Well-being for Desk Dwellers and Couch Potatoes)

PJ Sharon

PJ SHARON

All rights reserved. Except for use in any review, or as permitted under the U.S. Copyright Act of 1976, no part of this publication may be reproduced, distributed, or transmitted in any form or by any means, or stored in a database or retrieval system, without prior written permission of the author. This e-book is licensed for your personal enjoyment only. This e-book may not be re-sold or given away to other people. If you would like to share this book with another person, please purchase an additional copy for each recipient. If you're reading this book and did not purchase it, or it was not purchased for your use only, then please return to your retailer and purchase your own copy. Thank you for respecting the hard work of this author.

Note to reader:

This publication contains the opinions and ideas of its author. It is intended to provide helpful and informative material on the subjects addressed in the publication. The recommendations described herein are meant to supplement, and not to be a substitute for, professional medical care or treatment. It is sold with the understanding that the author and publisher are not engaged in rendering medical, health, or any other kind of professional services in the book. The reader should consult his or her medical, health, or other competent professional before adopting any of the suggestions in this book or drawing inferences from it. The author and publisher specifically disclaim all responsibility for any liability, loss, or risk, personal or otherwise, which is incurred as a consequence, directly or indirectly, of the use and application of any of the contents of this book.

Cover by The Killion Group

Stock Photos via Deposit Photos and Big Stock Photos

Photography by Sally Ames Vaillancourt

Edited by Judy Roth

Copyright © 2016 PJ Sharon

All rights reserved.

ISBN: 10:1519110502
ISBN-13:978-1519110503

DEDICATION

For my clients and writer pals suffering the ravages of
Sedentary Lifestyle Syndrome.
Take heart, there is hope.

Lives are changed one choice at a time.

I also dedicate this book to my yoga students, who keep me grounded and give me another reason to come down from
my mountain.
I appreciate each and every one of you.

CONTENTS

Acknowledgments

    Introduction   7

1. Understanding Your Body   9
2. Prevention   15
3. Pain Management   20
4. Choosing Your Health Care Team   26
5. Fighting the Battle of the Bulge   32
6. Metabolic Syndrome   43
7. Importance of Sleep   50
8. Ergonomics 101   54
9. Exercise Basics   62
10. Stretching Exercises   68
11. Strengthening Exercises   98
12. Treatment and Self Care   121
13. Stress Management 101   146
14. Making or Breaking a Habit   157
15. Tips for Special Groups   165
16. PJ's Snack Healthy Tips & Smoothie Recipes   175

    Final Note   184

    About the Author   185

    Other Books by PJ Sharon   186

Stevie,
To your best health in 2016!

R Sloan

ACKNOWLEDGMENTS

First and foremost, thank you to my clients, friends, and professional contacts who encouraged me to write this book. They've told me it's long overdue. I hope this is what you had in mind. Otherwise, I might have to write another. For now, this should tide you over.

The final product would not be what it is without my fabulous photographer friend, Sally Vaillincourt, whose generosity and enthusiasm for this project brings tears to my eyes. Thanks for your patience, perseverance, and vision. I want to also thank Linda Pollock, owner of Back in Touch Wellness in East Granby, CT., for being my model on this project and for supporting me in countless ways. You're as beautiful on the inside as you are on the outside.

To my social media friends on Facebook, Twitter, and around the cyber-sphere, thanks for spreading the love. Title credit goes to Bill and Katy Lee, and thanks to Kim Gorman for help with the tag line, "Stand up for your life!" Brilliant!

I'd like to add a huge shout out to my writer friends, who are the most amazing group of generous, creative, dynamic, and hardest working people I've ever met. You all rock and I couldn't do this without you.

A special thanks to my beta readers Christine Wunch, Corinna Lawson, and Joy Smith, and my editor on this project, Judy Roth. You make me work hard for it, but the final draft is always worth the effort. Thanks for pushing me to do my best. You helped put the shine on it.

Last, but most certainly not least, thank you to my wonderfully patient and talented husband, aka, the "tech-spert." I would be hopelessly lost without your love, support, and encouragement. You are the best man I've ever known.

INTRODUCTION

I often ask my friends in the writing community, "Is your writing killing you?" They know me well enough to realize that I am only half joking. But for those of you who suffer from **"Sedentary Lifestyle Syndrome,"** hereby known as **SLS**, you understand completely. If you spend hours a day at your desk or in your car, or find yourself imprisoned by your computers and perpetually attached to your cell phones, iPads and e-readers, you know the pitfalls of the sedentary and chair-bound lifestyle all too well. Do you suffer neck and back pain, poor posture, symptoms of carpal tunnel syndrome, or even significant weight gain from all the sitting you do? With today's fast paced, digitized world, we're all finding ourselves in this predicament and there seems to be no end in sight to the perils of techno-overload and the inevitable decline of our health as a result.

Leading researchers in the medical community are claiming that "sitting is the new smoking." Research shows that prolonged sitting increases your risk for cancer, heart disease, obesity, Type 2 Diabetes, and even depression. James Levine, a Mayo Clinic endocrinologist and researcher, says obese people sit on average two-and-a-half hours more every day than thinner people. If that's not enough reason to get up off the couch or move away from your desk every half hour, I challenge you to find your own "WHY." What will it take for you to make a change right now? Do you want to see your children and grandchildren grow up? Do you want to fit into that closet full of clothes that have somehow "shrunk" while on the hanger? One of the many great lessons I've learned from fitness guru, Jillian Michaels, is to find your "WHY." Reminding yourself of *why* you're fighting to get fit when the going gets tough will give you the strength to overcome any challenge you might face with the "HOW."

This book was written for all of you writers, readers, desk dwellers, and self-proclaimed couch potatoes out there. In this practical guide, I'll help you understand your body and your pain, and its relationship to posture, bio-mechanics, and ergonomics (the study of human capabilities in relation to work demands—or, to simplify for our purposes—workstation setup). I'll offer simple, easy to implement suggestions for improving your workstation, dietary tips to combat what I call, "the sitter's spread," and exercises to prevent and alleviate common orthopedic conditions that result from prolonged sitting, poor posture, and faulty ergonomics.

With over twenty-five years in the health and fitness profession, first as a Physical Therapist Assistant, and then as a Licensed Massage Therapist, personal trainer, and yoga instructor, I have learned the skills it takes to maintain my own health and well-being while working as a full time writer and business owner. I won't lie and say it's easy, or that I don't have my struggles. We all do! But the information I'll share with you in this book will give you a solid foundation and the tools you need to effectively care for yourself and take control of your body, your health, and your life.

If you think I don't understand your suffering, think again. I live with, and manage, chronic pain every day. After years of abusing my body with sports, car accidents, and repetitive traumas, my spine is unstable. Ligaments that hold my spine and pelvis together have become over stretched, causing daily occurrences of misalignment. Thank goodness I know how to fix it when my neck or low back "go out."

Short of fusing my spine (not an option since I'm functional and healthy), or treating me with pain meds (also not an option—by my choice), there isn't much that Western Medicine can do for me. X-rays show that I have arthritis (Degenerative Joint Disease) and bone spurs in my neck and back, and with the amount of sitting/writing I do, it's an uphill battle to live pain-free and med-free, keep my weight under control, and wear a happy smile every day. But at 51 years-old and a grandmother, I can still drop and do twenty-five push-ups, stand on my head, and heft 40 pound bags of pellets into my pellet stove when old man winter comes calling. I exercise regularly, eat relatively healthy, and take daily supplements and natural remedies, but nothing narcotic for pain management.

The tips I've included in this book can get you to that level of functional fitness in spite of your struggle to sit up straight at the computer or the chronic pain in the neck that isn't your aunt Josephine. (I have no cure for pesky relatives.)

I've treated hundreds of clients over the years who have benefited from the helpful advice and simple, life-changing tips I'll share with you in the following chapters. I'll guide you through choosing your health-care team and give you simple exercises you can do—even at your desk.

Testimonial:

As a writer and a publicist, I spend a lot of time sitting at my computer. After learning and following the simple stretching and ergonomics lessons taught by Ms. Sharon, I have less tension and can work for longer periods of time without painful interruption.
Jennifer F. (Author and publicist)

Included in the book are my best, stay slim secrets, quick-fix stretches, and ways to adjust your workstation set up, "MacGyver" style. I've even included a few of my favorite smoothie and snack recipes to help keep you healthy and energized while you're writing that novel, caught up in a reading marathon, or embarking on that cross country road trip. So read on, write on, and take control of your health today. Don't wait for your writing—or your sedentary lifestyle—to kill you.

Stand up for your life!

CHAPTER 1

UNDERSTANDING YOUR BODY

Fabulous! You've taken the first step by opening this book and diving in. That tells me you're serious about making some changes and optimizing your health. Before we get to all the good stuff, let's start with the basics. Understanding how your body works, how it moves, and how you can gain control of it, is the first step toward creating the best you that you can be. No worries; this won't be an anatomy lesson or another boring "how to" book. I'll be sharing with you all the helpful tips I give my massage patients, personal training clients, and yoga students every day. Hopefully, you'll find the information easy to understand and equally as easy to implement into your daily life. Let's get started.

If you've been living a sedentary lifestyle, you're probably also living with some amount of pain or discomfort. What is pain? The Oxford Dictionary defines it as *physical discomfort caused by injury or illness; mental suffering*. This is an overly simplistic definition, but one we can all relate to. If you've had pain—and let's face it; we've all felt pain at one time or another, and many of us live with it on a daily basis—you know that it can definitely affect us mentally and emotionally, as well as physically. Physical pain weakens us. Perhaps only temporarily with an acute injury. But what about the effects of chronic pain brought on by overuse injuries, poor postural awareness, and the day-to-day abuses we inflict upon ourselves under the guise of suffering for our craft and living in this fast-paced, computer-driven society? Depending upon our tolerance and fortitude, physical pain can be nothing more than a nuisance. Or…it can derail our plans faster than you can say, *pass the pain pills*. In addition, the mental/emotional toll of pain shouldn't be dismissed. Chronic pain can lead to depression and anxiety, sending us spiraling downward into a debilitating cycle.

I'll note here the difference between acute and chronic pain. In this text, we'll mostly be dealing with the chronic variety.

Without getting into neuro-anatomy and physiology, the pain response is the body's primitive defense mechanism—an involuntary neurological response that produces a reflexive retraction from the painful stimulus. Thanks to this reflexive response, we naturally have a tendency to protect the body from further harm, and we become conditioned to avoid future painful encounters. If you've been burned on a hot stove, you won't want to put your hands near the burner again.

Acute pain happens when you injure soft tissues, joints, bones, or muscles—usually in response to a direct stimulus, such as with touching a hot stove or stubbing a toe. It is generally immediate, of short duration, and the injury heals over time, allowing you to return to full function. In more severe cases, acute pain may be a result of serious or even life threatening conditions. Falls, car accidents, and organ malfunctions such as appendicitis or cardiac events are categorized as acute. Often, these acute conditions require treatment, rehabilitation, or other intervention to restore full function, but within a relatively short period of time, your pain dissipates and is soon forgotten.

Chronic pain, on the other hand, sticks around. Pain may come on slowly and become progressively worse due to degenerative diseases like arthritis, degenerative disc disease, or neurological disorders such as Parkinson's, Multiple Sclerosis, or Anterolateral Sclerosis (ALS). Other chronic pain inducers are less easily diagnosed but just as debilitating. Complex conditions, such as fibromyalgia or chronic fatigue syndrome, which have underlying and often misdiagnosed symptomology, can leave sufferers feeling frustrated and alone in their pain, since they are often made to feel as if, *it's all in their head.*

Depression and mental illness can also lead to chronic pain symptoms, and may even be secondary consequences of living with chronic pain. With these long term and less obvious contributors, chronic pain can be complicated to treat. If you suffer from chronic pain, it's important to seek advice from your doctor about various treatments, both traditional and alternative (including acupuncture, massage therapy, physical therapy, or chiropractic/osteopathic intervention). Medication may help, but just as likely, lifestyle changes become necessary to manage or overcome the condition.

Some might say, *your pain is telling you something*. But what exactly is our pain telling us? And how can we learn to listen and adapt our lifestyle to alleviate it? Yes. Not just live with it, learn to cope, suck it up, or "manage" it. In many cases, you can alleviate your pain entirely. There are no guarantees, but if you're willing to make changes—to take positive steps—one after another, you can most definitely improve the quality of your life.

Basics of posture, alignment, and biomechanics

The type of chronic pain we'll be addressing here is categorized as Overuse Syndrome, Repetitive Strain, or Biomechanical Pain Syndrome. These conditions are brought on by muscle imbalances caused by repetitive stresses to the musculoskeletal system, either through poor posture/biomechanics or inappropriate workstation set-up. Over time, and without intervention, destruction to soft tissues and improper spinal alignment can lead to severe and debilitating health issues. Living with this type of chronic pain makes it nearly impossible to consistently function at a high level, accomplish the goals we set for ourselves, or achieve our dreams.

On the upside, we can do something about it.

Correct Posture

Let's look for a moment at how our bodies work. Again, for the purposes of this text, I'll simplify matters by leaving out the gritty details of the nervous system's information super highway and focus on the fundamentals of the musculoskeletal system. Stay with me for this short anatomy lesson and don't let the technical stuff scare you off. The important thing is that you have a general idea of the workings of your spine and how it supports your framework.

Our musculoskeletal system is comprised of:
- An **axial skeleton** (our spine, which is made up of 7 cervical, 12 thoracic, and 5 lumbar vertebrae, as well as a pelvis and sacrum)
- An **appendicular skeleton** (appendages, or limbs)
- And the **ligaments, tendons, and muscles** (I'll include the soft tissue and fascial system here) that hold it all together.

The **musculoskeletal system** as a whole is an intricate system of pulleys, hinges, ball and socket and gliding joints, and the puppet strings that make them move—muscles, tendons, and ligaments.

The **fascial system** is a web of connective tissue that runs through your entire body. Picture taking the skin off a piece of raw chicken. The white, filmy, fibrous material you see woven throughout the muscle and covering the outside is called fascia. We have this same system of connective tissue that runs throughout the entire body from head to toe in a continuous web. With inactivity, injury, illness, or just plain lack of lubrication, this web of connective tissue can become more fibrous, bind down, and adhere to surrounding tissues, further restricting movement and causing a myriad of problems we are just beginning to understand.

When all is in correct working order, the muscles are balanced, the fascia is without restriction, and the spine remains in proper alignment for optimal function.

We call this *neutral* position. Imagine though, the consequences of sitting all day in front of a computer screen—a position we are clearly not made to remain in for extended periods of time. The weight of our head on our shoulders—as our eyes focus on the task before us—draws us slightly forward. Our natural inclination is to keep our eyes level and steady on our screen, so as we allow our shoulders to round, our head to tilt back, and our chin to jut out—our spinal alignment is compromised from the cervical spine down to our tailbone. No more neutral position.

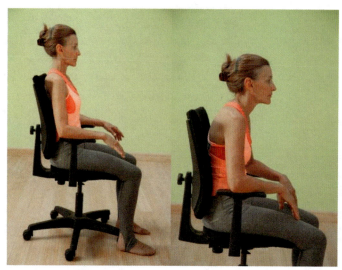

Fig. 1 Correct Posture   **Fig. 2 Incorrect Posture**

In response to this *__forward head posture__*, the posterior cervical muscles shorten and become tighter as the anterior muscles lengthen and become weaker. With our hands on the keyboard and mouse, gravity and the weight of our arms in front of us cause our shoulders to round forward, shortening our chest wall and anterior shoulder muscles and lengthening/weakening our scapular retractors in the upper back, which are designed to hold us upright. We lose the natural lumbar curve in the lower spine and we find ourselves sitting on our tailbone rather than our ischial tuberosities, or "sit" bones.

This loss of structure—over time—leads to muscle imbalances, fascial restrictions, stresses on the discs and vertebral bodies (eventually leading to degenerative joint disease, arthritis, and spurring of the bones), and weakness of core stabilizers that keep our spine aligned properly. This is the perfect set up for chronic pain to develop. Remember when we said that your pain is trying to tell you something? Well, this is it.

Correct your posture!

I know…I'm over simplifying the problem and realize it's an uphill battle, but one well worth fighting. Consider this. Your head weighs between eight and twelve pounds (depending on how big your brain is or how hard-headed you are). Relatively, it's about as big as a bowling ball. If you hold a ten pound bowling ball in close to your chest, it doesn't weigh that much, but extend it six or eight-inches out in front of you and try to hold it there, and you'll get an idea of how much harder your neck and upper back muscles have to work to keep your head on your shoulders when you aren't in good posture.

The same is true for your lower back. That's why bending at the knees and hips is so important when lifting.

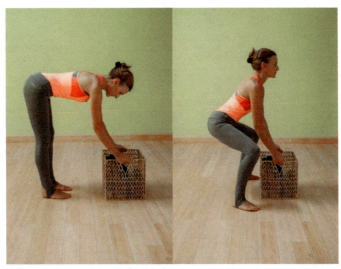

Fig. 4 Incorrect Lifting   Fig. 5 Correct Lifting

The average force to your lumbar spine when you bend forward with your legs straight is about 400 pounds of pressure (again…depending on your size and weight). If you consider your sacrum your center of gravity (fulcrum), and begin to lean forward without bending your knees, you have to multiply the weight of your upper body times the angle you create when your shoulders move beyond your toes. The further out you lean without bending your knees, the more pressure you place on the low back. Think about that the next time you bend to lift that laundry basket or box of books.

Understanding how the body works and moves is essential in correcting bad habits. We can learn to protect ourselves by changing how we move, moderating the stresses we place on our bodies, and being mindful of maintaining a neutral spine whenever possible. This awareness alone will go a long way toward keeping you pain free and healthy for the duration of your sitting career. An excellent resource for gaining knowledge in the area of movement re-education is the **Alexander Technique.**

The Alexander Technique (AT) was developed in the early 20th century before ergonomics became a recognized science and has been applied since then by people of all ages and professions. The technique can be described as a simple and practical educational method that alerts people to ways in which they are misusing their bodies, and how their everyday habits of work may be harming them. It teaches people how to avoid habits that create excessive amounts of static work and how to reduce the amount of unnecessary muscular force they are applying to their bodies. Stated another way, the Alexander Technique teaches the use of the appropriate amount of effort for a particular activity. Check online for more information about AT and where you might find a practicing therapist near you. http://www.ergonomics.org/

You might also consider consulting a physical therapist who practices the Feldenkrais method, another type of movement reeducation program, consisting of a series of exercises designed to restructure your movement patterns and correct imbalances. I use these principles in my practice with good results. Check online for therapists in your area.

Realize that you'll never be able to keep perfect posture all the time or move without a few missteps in proper body mechanics, but if you can be more aware even 25-50% of the time, think of the benefits and the reduction

in wear and tear on your body. It might be as simple as:
- Setting a timer every 30-60 minutes and doing a few stretches before continuing your work.
- Or getting up frequently to do some standing activities.
- Try writing in sprints. I usually take a ten to fifteen minute break at least every hour. I'll either stretch, do a load of laundry or dishes, or take a short walk. Then it's back to work for another 30-60 minute sprint.

This gets harder when you're on a deadline or only have a small window of opportunity to work, but as soon as you sense your posture degrading, that's your signal to get up and move. For some of us, that means every 30 minutes. **Don't wait until you're in pain!**

NOTE: There are some great apps to help you keep track of screen time. You can go old school and set a kitchen timer or download an app that will remind you to move when your thirty minutes or hour is up. I like the Stay Focused app for my Android phone, but your Fitbit Charge or any basic stop watch type timer will do in a pinch. http://www.online-stopwatch.com/loop-countdown/. **For Mac users there's an app called Time Out** (http://www.dejal.com/timeout/) **that will remind you to take breaks, offer soothing musical selections, or signal micro breaks every ten minutes so you can check in to make sure your posture is up to snuff. There are several other online timer apps that work on most operating systems, or you can invest in a program called the Pomodoro Technique** http://pomodorotechnique.com/ **that trains you to organize your work into 25 minute segments. It's said to increase productivity as well as improve work/life balance.**

More on work/life balance in the chapter on **STRESS MANAGEMENT 101.** For now, I only want you to recognize one thing. It's time for you to stand up for your life…literally and figuratively. You are the only one who can make the necessary changes to improve your health and the quality of your life. It begins with awareness, and now that you're aware of why prolonged sitting is causing problems, it's up to you to do something about it.

CHAPTER 2

PREVENTION

Let's say you're a newbie at the sedentary lifestyle thing. You've avoided getting sucked into social media, gaming, driving an hour to work each way, sitting for hours staring at a computer screen, or otherwise abusing your body by hanging out in all the wrong places. Right? You exercise four or five times a week, take the stairs instead of the elevator, and you eat your veggies and drink your eight glasses of water daily. Kudos! Prevention for you is easy. Keep those healthy habits and you'll be golden.

But give into the bad habits of poor posture and sedentary living, and over time, the effects will creep up on you before you can say *Ouch!* You'll start to put on a few pounds, notice more frequent headaches, maybe a stiff neck or sore shoulders, and then…bam! What is that tingling in my hands, and why am I waking up in the morning and crawling out of bed like a tin man with rusty hinges?

It might be five years or ten years down the road, but trust me, adopting unhealthy habits now will catch up with you eventually. Once the damage to joints is done and muscle imbalances abound, you'll likely end up in the **pain management** group. We can't control everything, but the choices we make today affect us tomorrow. It's that simple…and that complicated. Car accidents happen. Falls happen. Life happens. Genetics and family dynamics influence who we are and how we make choices in our everyday lives. And as hard as we try to be good, inevitably someone brings chocolate or doughnuts—or chocolate doughnuts—into the office, and we are caught in a moment of weakness.

Although prevention in this case is worth several pounds of cure, there is only so much we can do to combat the stress on the body that is inflicted by eight-plus hours a day at our computers and workstations. Students are required to sit in class all day and then study at night, full time employees are responsible for meeting quotas, and editors have firm deadlines. Even as an author, I work under tremendous pressure to finish the next book, and spend hours a day on promotion and marketing. But here's the thing. It comes down to choices. As with most things in life, we can choose to give in to what's easy, or we can choose to do what is in our best interest. Hiding from reality isn't going to make the hard stuff go away. That chocolate is still going to be there, and it is still up to us to say no. Suddenly prevention doesn't seem so easy.

I'll go back to what I said before. You can't be perfect all the time but think in percentages. If I eat the right foods eighty percent of the time, it won't kill me to eat a nice piece of dark chocolate now and then—or even a doughnut. Gorging on a whole box of bonbons or munchkins? Not okay. Take one. Savor it. Chew it twenty times before swallowing. Drink a glass of water afterwards and go find something else to do besides stare at the box longingly on the countertop. Or move them out of your vision entirely. Better yet, tell your spouse, co-workers, or employees to knock off the sweets at the office and recommend rotating turns and each bringing a healthy snack once a week. Start a walking group at lunch time. Buddy up and ask for support in your weight loss and activity goals. Be proactive about your health and support those around you to be the healthiest they can be. You'll be surprised by who will join in.

In the office: If you have people working for you, you know the benefits of having a healthy crew. You hired these people. You owe it to yourself and them to provide a safe and healthy work environment. Healthy employees mean less absenteeism, higher productivity, improved morale, and workers with positive mental attitudes. Office workers are competitive people. Start a monthly challenge and award small prizes for your employees.

- A five dollar Amazon or B&N gift card or movie tickets would suffice to show you care and value their efforts.
- Reward them for the little things and keep it fun. Give an award for most push-ups or sit-ups, most steps for the month for Fitbit users, or give incentives for creative ways to boost productivity while boosting a healthy office lifestyle.
- Create an exercise space at work. It doesn't take much room to house a mat, some resistive bands, and a physio-ball.
- Allow people who choose to exercise to have an extra fifteen minutes at lunch time.
- Limit unhealthy foods at the office by starting a healthy snack club.

For my writer pals out there, writers in online groups love to do word-count oriented writing sprints. Why not add a physical component and suggest twenty-five wall push-ups or ten squats for every thousand words written? You get the picture. Prevention is about getting in front of the problem. Here is a short list of things you can do today to improve the quality of your life and health, reduce your risk of injury, and curtail illness. There will be more about each tip later in the book.

Stay hydrated. I cannot stress enough the importance of keeping your body hydrated. Without proper hydration, every system in your body will be compromised and unable to work optimally. Cells need water, muscles need water, your organs need water, and yes, your brain needs water. A quick formula for proper water intake is your weight in pounds, divided by three. That's the minimum of how many ounces of water you should drink each day. A 150 pound woman should drink approximately 50 ounces of water, whereas a 210 pound male should drink upwards of 70 ounces of water per day—minimum. Some fitness gurus suggest half your weight in ounces. Although the old idea of eight, 8-oz glasses of water per day (a whopping 64 ounces) is considered the gold standard, it makes sense that the individual build of the person and the type of activity the person does on a routine basis should be taken into account.

Proper hydration is the #1 weight management tool I recommend to my clients.

Fill a 24 ounce water bottle first thing in the morning and keep it with you. (Sure, give it a name and treat it like a pal.) As a bonus calorie burner, make it ice water. Your body has to burn more calories warming the water to body temperature. Just be prepared to carry an extra sweater and know where the nearest restrooms are at all times.

As an aside, alcohol, soda (diet or otherwise), and caffeinated products don't count—at least in my book. These are dehydrating substances that will ultimately sap your energy and leave you feeling depleted rather than renewed. Not that you can't have your morning coffee or afternoon tea, and an occasional glass of wine in the evening; just don't count them toward your hydration goal. You can count vitamin waters and juices as long as they aren't laden with sugar or artificial sweeteners. If they are, water them down. Or you can make your own flavored drinks by adding lemon or fresh berries to your water for a tasty refreshing drink. Agave, stevia, honey, or coconut sugar are healthier options for sweetening than refined and processed sugars or artificial sweeteners, but avoid adding any type of sugar if you can.

Get Moving. This probably goes without saying, but the more you can add movement into your daily routine, the better off you are. The general consensus is that **for every hour you spend at the computer or sitting, you need ten minutes of exercise to combat the effects.** If you want to stand up, jog in place, do jumping jacks, sit-ups, and push-ups every hour for ten minutes, great! For me, it translates to thirty minutes of vigorous exercise five times per week, and several mini stretch breaks during my work day. If a half hour commitment four to five times per week is asking too much, the stretches I'll give you later in this book will easily fill those hourly ten minute breaks with great tools to keep your body healthier and happier than it's been in years. Honestly, though, you can do ANYTHING for thirty minutes a day. You're worth it. Your health is worth it. Feeling great and being fit…is worth thirty minutes, no matter how busy you are. The only person preventing you from taking time for your health is YOU.

A NOTE on OVERCOMING INERTIA: During a massage session one of my clients presented the challenge of *overcoming inertia* as being her biggest stumbling block to regular exercise. She explained it as an inability to find the motivation to get up off her butt. Others have expressed this same idea, lamenting that if they could only be like a wind-up doll or the energizer bunny armed with some external motivator that would get them going, they could do it. It made me think about Parkinson's sufferers who often experience a sense of being "frozen" in mid movement. No matter how hard they try, their feet will remain glued to the floor until enough messages are sent to the brain or some external stimulus triggers their neurons to fire and their muscles to jump to action. Sometimes it takes something as small as a gentle push from a caregiver or a line drawn on the floor ahead of them on which they can focus, to get them moving again, but they will tell you, until that switch is turned on, they are "stuck".

That's how most of us feel. No matter how much we want to move forward and make healthier choices, something stops us. We feel helpless to overcome our own inertia and until that switch is thrown we stay stuck. If I had the magic bullet to solve this problem, I would surely be a billionaire. But the truth is, whatever motivates a person to take charge of his or her life and make necessary changes, is different for everyone.

I can tell you that external motivators, like fitting into a wedding dress or dropping a few pounds for that class reunion coming up are only temporarily effective. You might be able to deprive yourself or drastically change your eating habits for a short time to meet a single goal, but lifelong changes require new patterns of thinking that will lead to new patterns of behavior—which will ultimately help you achieve your goals and stick to a plan. We all know that the immediate gratification of eating that donut is more powerful in the moment than any short term, temporary goal. External motivators are seen as something out in the future and will likely take a back seat to our sugar addiction and need for comfort when we're stressed.

Internal motivators, however, are the most powerful catalysts for change. How badly do you want to be fit and healthy? WHY do you want it? And what are you willing to do to achieve it? Internal motivators like wanting to feel better about ourselves, have a sexy body, or set a good example for our children are usually longer term and more powerful motivations because they have longer reaching effects and have a greater perceived intrinsic value. It doesn't mean you won't fall back into old habits, but the stronger your internal motivation is for WHY you want to be active, fit, and healthy, the more likely you will keep coming back to making healthier choices on a regular basis. Like the Parkinson's sufferer, sometimes it takes a nudge from outside ourselves, and sometimes it's just a matter of keeping our eyes focused on the goal before us to break through that state of inertia.

Motivational speaker Harv Ecker says, "Do what's easy and life will be hard, but do what's hard, and life will be easy." He has a point. Each time you stay focused on your WHY, choose to do the right thing, make the hard decision, or force yourself to overcome inertia, the new pattern of behavior will be reinforced. The payoff is being one step closer to your goals. I'm not saying that making the right choices is ever going to be easy, but the long term benefits are so worth the effort that I guarantee you won't regret skipping that donut.

Modify your workstation. I'll give you more details on this throughout the book and specifically in the **ERGONOMICS** section, but if you're having pain from being at your desk too long, or God forbid, you're still sitting on the couch working on your laptop, make a change…NOW! Nothing is more important to the longevity of your writing/sitting career than providing a safe and properly designed workstation for yourself. If sitting is killing you, try a standing desk, a treadmill desk, or cycle your way through your inbox with a Fit Desk.

Learn to dictate your notes into a recorder and transcribe them later in manageable pieces when you can sit properly at your desktop computer. Dragon software and other voice recording systems might be exactly what you need to increase productivity while reducing wear and tear on your body. Whatever reason you have for martyring yourself and suffering through the pain, figure it out and get over it. **Hurting yourself helps no one!** I'll give you some practical tips later on how to MacGyver your setup if money is tight and you're looking for shortcuts.

Make stretching part of your life every day. In the shower, in the car, at your desk, or even standing in the grocery store line, there are simple stretches you can incorporate into your day that will help minimize your pain and ensure your muscles stay strong and flexible for life. The stretches in this book are meant to fit the bill.

I highly recommend taking a gentle yoga class a couple of times a week if you can. Yoga integrates whole body movement. It incorporates stretching, strengthening, stabilizing, and balance activities that can not only leave you feeling longer, leaner, and more relaxed, but can even heal the body on many levels. Remember, I spoke earlier of the importance of awareness of how we move? Yoga is a wonderful teacher. It trains us to be mindful and present in our bodies, teaches us to breathe, and can reduce our toxic stress by improving the circulation of our bodily fluids and opening the energy channels where we often have blockages due to stagnation, injury, or illness.

Make your health your #1 priority. I pointed out above that hurting yourself helps no one. Here's the hard truth. You are ultimately responsible for your health and well-being, so it's up to you to gather the tools you need to make informed decisions about diet, nutrition, exercise, and living a balanced life. Educate yourself.

There are hundreds of thousands of websites, magazines, and books about these topics. Yes, you have to weed through some misinformation and be discriminating about what you integrate into your life, but let common sense be your guide. The bottom line is that if you don't take care of yourself, no one else will do it for you, so take the time to learn HOW to take care of yourself.

Get regular screenings such as mammograms, pap-smears, a colonoscopy at age fifty, prostate exams, and even regular eye and dental check-ups.

Early detection of disease leads to early treatment and increased survival rates. Treat yourself to a massage once a month or as often as you can afford it and don't feel guilty about taking time for yourself. Whatever you do, don't ignore your health maintenance duties. **Denial is not your friend.** These are important preventative measures that allow you to live a healthy, productive life. You must know by now that you can't effectively care for anyone else unless you first take care of yourself.

Stop making excuses. I'm going to take a moment to be harsh, and it's only because I love you and want what's best for you. My comments are based on my own life experience and what I believe to be true. Don't take it personally or let your ego jump to your rescue by sticking your fingers in your ears and loudly saying la-la-la. Listen up.

Unless you are literally dying, you have no excuse to be lazy, overweight, unmotivated, or whiney. And even if you are dying…you don't want to waste one minute of your best life because you decided to wallow. We all have bad days, and it's okay to give in to tears or the occasional pity party, but then I suggest you suck it up, take a breath, wipe the tears away, and get back up on the damn horse.

I know how hard life can be. I meet people in my work every day who are in really rough shape. Some—even dying. The ones who are happiest, healthiest, and most at peace, even when their bodies are ready to give out, are the ones who stand up and fight. They don't make excuses for why they can't do something. They focus on the things they can do and avoid staying "stuck." They look for the positives, the beauty in the little things, and the power of living in the moment. If they can do it, so can you.

I understand the debilitating nature of depression and mental illness and the impact that these conditions can have on chronic pain and maintaining a positive mental attitude. But even people who suffer from mental illness have choices. They can seek help, ask for support, and manage their illness with grace and dignity if they so choose. One day at a time…one choice at a time.

CHAPTER 3

PAIN MANAGEMENT

If you are a sedentary lifestyle expert you are likely already familiar with chronic pain and have been working to manage it. Pain management can feel like Aunt Josephine has moved in full time, and there is no end in sight. So how do we learn to live with it?

Pain management is, once again, often about choices. You're no doubt familiar with over the counter anti-inflammatory medications like Advil (Ibuprophen) and Aleve (naproxen). These NSAIDS (non-steroidal anti-inflammatory drugs) can be a life saver for the occasional headache or muscle/joint pains inherent with living in these earth-suits we call bodies. Even Tylenol (acetaminophen), Excedrin (combination of acetaminophen, aspirin, and caffeine), or other over the counter pain relievers can take the edge off. However, it's been shown that consistent use of these products can lead to stomach ulcers, liver and kidney toxicity, and a host of other issues that will do nothing to "cure" your pain. These are at best, palliative in nature, offering temporary relief. Of course, this is only one aspect of pain management—and not my favorite approach, although many people have found temporary and even long-term relief from properly prescribed and well monitored medications.

For the chronic pain sufferer, stronger medications may be necessary. Site injections, nerve blocks, or even surgical intervention might be on the horizon if the pain persists and becomes intolerable.

If you suffer chronic pain, talk with your physician and decide together what plan is right for you.

You may have gathered by now that I'm a fan of alternative medicine. More specifically, I prefer to approach illness and injury from a broader perspective, which means **integrating** traditional Western Medicine with Eastern Medicine philosophies and holistic health practices. This is, by definition, what **Integrative Medicine** is all about. I don't believe that one is better than the other as much as I think they both offer a great deal of help and hope when used in combination.

Let me give you a common scenario I've seen again and again in my years of practice. Take, for instance, that numbness and tingling in your hands we talked about. The condition has developed over time and there has been no specific accident or injury that brought it on. Symptoms are worse when you're at your computer, driving, or when you first wake up in the morning. You seek out your primary care physician (PCP), who, if he or she (I'll say "he" for our example) is good with a quick differential diagnosis, determines that your symptoms are likely caused from a pinched nerve brought on by poor posture and repetitive strain. He gives you a prescription for an anti-inflammatory ("a therapeutically effective" dose at 800 milligrams, to be taken as many as three times a day. If you're lucky, he or your pharmacist reminds you to take it with food). He tells you if your symptoms don't improve in six weeks, to come back and see him. After a few days on the meds, the pain is significantly reduced—hallelujah—but now your stomach feels as if you've swallowed glass from taking the mega doses of anti-inflammatories, so you decide to cut back.

Long story short, your symptoms return and you end up back at the doctor's office six weeks later. He will likely recommend some prescription antacid to go with your anti-inflammatory, or perhaps offer a stronger pain medication at this point. Or he'll send you to an orthopedist for a cortisone injection if your tendons in the shoulder or at the elbow are screaming their contribution. The orthopedist—if he's worth his salt—will do an X-ray, find nothing earth shattering, give you a miraculously pain relieving shot, and recommend that you wear wrist braces when you sleep, type, or do anything requiring lifting or repetitive movement. He tells you to come back in six weeks if you aren't better.

You get great relief (if you're lucky and compliant), but inevitably, a few months later your symptoms return and you go another round with the needle. Maybe the orthopedist sends you to physical therapy this time. This is a fabulous idea, and would have worked dandy if the PCP had sent you four months ago, because now you have a chronic condition that has had time to fester and cause damage to joints, nerves, and soft tissue structures. Give your pain a name because it's probably going to be around for a while. Let's call it Fred (after my crotchety old grandfather).

The physical therapists, if they are well-trained, insightful, and not seeing patients every twenty minutes, will likely do a thorough evaluation, often pinpointing the etiology (origin) of your symptoms and determining whether you actually have Carpal Tunnel Syndrome (CTS) or if the problem is coming from elsewhere, such as with Thoracic Outlet Syndrome (TOS)(where nerve entrapment in the brachial plexus or vascular compression is the culprit), or if perhaps a cervical disc bulge is causing the symptoms. Although physical therapists aren't generally able to make an official diagnosis and must rely on the doctors to be on top of things, their assessment usually uncovers a more specific differential diagnosis simply because they spend more hands on time with you and orthopedics is their specialty. A treatment plan is set up and you'll probably see the therapist two to three times per week for three to four weeks, depending on your insurance and how much you can afford in co-pays.

During that time, the therapist may try some calming modalities such as ultrasound, electrical stimulation, ionto or phonophoresis (using direct current electrical stimulation or ultrasound to drive medication into those inflamed tendon areas), and maybe some deep friction massage. If disc involvement is suspected, or alignment issues are contributing to your symptoms, gentle cervical traction and/or manual therapy is usually helpful.

The therapist will hopefully teach you some exercises to correct the muscle imbalances responsible for the underlying problems, help you with workstation suggestions, and recommend lifestyle modifications to reduce the stress on the body parts in question. As long as your insurance company doesn't restrict your visits or dictate what the therapist is allowed to do with you, six to ten weeks of PT—and compliance from you—might just fix the problem. A caveat here is that the inflammatory pain cycle is a tenacious beast and is easily triggered by familiar stimuli, so if you aren't super compliant with your exercises and self-care at home, or you do something risky like rake the lawn, vacuum the whole house, or go kayaking for a few hours, you probably haven't heard the last from Fred. It's also likely that if you don't address the source of the problem (repetitive stress), you might as well get Fred his own insurance plan because he's probably going to be with you for some time. You might even introduce him to Aunt Josephine.

If per chance, physical therapy doesn't solve the problem and you're back in the orthopedist's office a few months later, he may go through the whole process again or recommend surgery—which is often unnecessary and should always be a last resort.

Here's the thing. You've now spent six months and hundreds—maybe thousands—of dollars on deductibles, co-pays, and tests trying to figure this thing out, all the while living with numbness, pain, and daily limitations—when a few visits to a good physical therapist, massage therapist, chiropractor, osteopath, or acupuncturist may have done the trick early on. These "alternatives" may or may not be covered by your insurance and they aren't on the top of your PCP's tool box, so most people end up seeking out these treatment options on their own as a last resort, rather than incorporating them into their treatment plan from the start.

Don't be afraid to question your doctor and ask for what you need. He may meet your suggestion of trying physical therapy or massage therapy with a rousing, "Go for it!" Maybe, it just wasn't on his radar. If you have a doctor who isn't willing to trust your instincts about what you need, or one who refuses to work with you on an integrative approach, find a new doctor. There are more and more doctors who are open to this kind of relationship. In the long run, it makes their job easier if you're willing to be proactive and are trying to stay healthy. You might have to go through a few to find the right doc for you, but it's worth it to know you're both on the same page and that you can trust him to listen to you.

Penny wise, pound foolish?

I understand that you have to spend your health care dollars wisely—especially with the increase in out-of-pocket expenses these days, but let's go back to the idea of prevention. Wouldn't it be great if someone had actually observed your slumped posture and put their hands on your neck and shoulders when you first started developing symptoms, recognized that a pill wasn't going to "fix" the problem, and suggested some exercises, a change in your workstation, and a good massage right from the start? You might have spent a couple hundred dollars on a new chair, a wrist pad, and a foot rest, and an additional $70 an hour for a few sessions with a massage therapist, but you would have saved yourself months of pain, aggravation, lost productivity, and probably hundreds of dollars in healthcare costs. From where I stand, it comes down to being part of a trusted team, deciding on priorities, and getting the most bang for your buck.

Here's where I have to remind people that massage therapy is not just for relaxation, and it isn't only for the rich and famous. **STOP FEELING GUILTY FOR TAKING CARE OF YOURSELF!** For the cost of dinner and a movie once a month (or a daily Starbuck's caffe latte grande), you could have a massage, which over time, would have lasting and life-changing benefits. Here are several reasons everyone could benefit from having a massage on a regular basis.

- Reduces pain
- Increases mobility
- Promotes circulation
- Reduces stress and muscle tension
- Helps rid the body of toxins
- Contributes to a healthy immune system
- And promotes a sense of connection and well-being

And here are a few testimonials from my clients about how massage has changed their lives:

"The benefits of regular body work with PJ after my auto accident a few years ago have returned me to normal." **Paul D. (Retired Music Executive)**

"PJ's massages have made a huge difference in my life as I've weathered the aging process with arthritis." **Myrna R. (Voice Coach)**

"Through working with Ms. Sharon I've learned so much about the human anatomy and how it reacts to daily/job related activities, exercise, stress, pain and healing. Massage and exercises have helped me during my career as a painting contractor, and after abdominal and knee surgery. More importantly, I've learned how to recognize, treat and avoid trigger points that cause me pain." **Gina B. (Painting Contractor)**

"As a client of Ms. Sharon's for eight years, I look forward to every visit, as I always leave feeling lighter, taller and completely relaxed. My massage sessions have freed me from chronic neck pain and turned into a staple in my overall wellness regimen—the perfect way to rejuvenate after many high-intensity workouts." **Kristin H. (Commercial Communications Manager)**

In a world where we're constantly *disconnecting* from each other, and instead, finding ourselves plugged into our electronic devices—the long term effects of which are yet to be determined—massage should be a regular part of your wellness and health maintenance plan. If you can't afford once a month, try for every six weeks, or at the least, get seasonal tune-ups every three months. **You do it for your car. It's the least you can do for your body.** I'll tell you how to find a massage therapist who's right for you in the next section on **CHOOSING YOUR HEALTH CARE TEAM.**

More ways to take an integrated approach

I can assure you that acupuncture, even if you're terrified of needles, is NOT painful. I've found it incredibly helpful. For me, it relieves back and neck pain, works on lung and digestive issues, and even offered relief from my elbow tendonitis a few years ago. After acupuncture, it's not uncommon for me to sleep better, breathe better, and generally feel renewed. It constantly amazes me how everything in the body is related and how often I notice that things I didn't even know were bothering me, improve after acupuncture.

As for chiropractic care, I wasn't always a fan. I came from a physical therapy background and PT philosophies are often in conflict with the high velocity manipulation techniques employed by chiropractors and osteopaths. I was under the impression—and still question—whether manipulating patients who have chronic instability (such as I do), isn't going to promote even more instability over time. My intuition and my body tell me that this isn't the approach best suited for me. It stands to reason that with repeated adjustments requiring a forceful, quick stretch on already overstretched and weakened ligaments that the stability might degrade further. Others who have generally poor flexibility, tight ligaments and joints, and particularly "sticky" vertebrae that resist gentler methods, will sing the praises of regular chiropractic adjustments.

My views on chiropractic care softened several years ago when I met a young chiropractor who I hit it off with right away. We had surprisingly similar views on holistic health care, and I appreciated his multi-disciplinary approach to health and healing. He was open to my concerns about high velocity manipulation of the spine not being for everyone, and he agreed. He educated me on the alternatives, such as a "drop table" or use of an activator, a small mechanical device used to align the joints of the spine with minimal force. After a particularly bad episode with my back going out of alignment—where nothing I or my PT pals attempted fixed the problem—I gave in and asked him for help.

In one session, using the activator and a few gentle contract/relax techniques, he had me standing up straight and pain free for the first time in days. I was so impressed with the results of his holistic and gentle approach that I began leasing space in his office and building my massage practice next door. Whenever I couldn't "fix" my own back or neck, he was the first person I would seek out, and he quickly became a necessary member of my healthcare team.

I trust that you understand my point. There are "good" and "bad" practitioners in every profession, and not every modality is going to be right for you. Even in traditional medicine, someone has to graduate in the bottom half of the class, and a scalpel isn't always necessary when a skilled adjustment will do the trick.

There are many more treatment approaches lumped into the "alternative" health care realm, which I won't get into here, but I do recommend that you keep an open mind. As long as it won't hurt or hinder your recovery, give it a try. I've adopted aromatherapy and energy work into my seasonal cleansing routine as I find it works on deeper issues that I hold onto without realizing it. You shouldn't discount the necessity of treating your mind and spirit as well as your body. We are more than just the sum of our physical parts and should strive for a balanced approach to healing our whole being.

Homeopathy, cranio-sacral therapy, sound healing, yoga, meditation, and Reiki all have merit and can have positive effects on maintaining good health and treating injury and disease. The healing power of the mind and the gift of a healing touch can offer amazing results. Since it's difficult to measure data, and individual results (and practitioners) vary greatly, research is underfunded and often not prioritized because of low returns on profitability. In addition, serious misconceptions about alternative therapies as "quackery" have been perpetuated by medical professionals, pharmaceutical lobbies, and insurance companies afraid of losing business. Granted, there are some practitioners of alternative therapies that give the industry a bad name by promising "cures" for all that ails you or offering ineffective treatments that do nothing more than empty your pocket. As I pointed out, there is "good" and "bad" in every profession, but let's not throw the baby out with the bath water, and let's not be naïve about what's behind the money driven propaganda against alternative medicine.

What would become of doctors and pharmaceutical giants if people stayed healthy and didn't need them anymore? God forbid! Doctors rely on evidence-based medicine with predictable outcomes and therefore consider intuitive therapies less reliable. Alternative medicine and study of the energy system is barely covered in most medical schools and doctors aren't inclined to take the time to learn about it afterwards since the current model of Western Medicine education has been the standard for decades. Change is slow, but it's coming.

Nikola Tesla once said, "If you want to learn the secrets of the Universe, think in terms of energy, frequency, and vibration."

Even Albert Einstein understood the possibilities beyond the measurable when he said, "It is entirely possible that behind the perception of our senses, worlds are hidden of which we are unaware."

I believe he and Mr. Tesla understood a fundamental truth that many medical practitioners miss. When we learn to rely on both science and nature equally, and respect the proven practices of other cultures, then we'll surely find the best of what medicine can offer.

Integrative medicine is growing in popularity, but the divide between traditional and alternative medicine philosophies still exist so don't expect your PCP to jump on board if he isn't already versed in alternative medicine theory. People are afraid of what they don't understand or aren't familiar with. As with anything you choose to incorporate into your health maintenance plan, you need to be your own advocate first and foremost. Do the research, be open minded, ask friends and trusted providers for recommendations, deal with budgetary limitations, and then choose what's right for you.

CHAPTER 4

CHOOSING YOUR HEALTH CARE TEAM

Ideally, your Primary Care Physician (PCP) should be your go to person for health care advice. They've spent years learning about the body and practicing the science of medicine. They are most informed about the latest drug therapies, testing procedures to help with proper diagnoses, and they are the people who will best direct you toward health and healing.

But here's the thing. The reality is, insurance industry requirements, liability costs, and the high price of medicine have crippled our medical community. It's extremely challenging to effectively practice not just the science of medicine but the art of medicine as well. As I mentioned before, treating the body, or—in this compartmentalized world of western medicine—treating only body parts, is going to lead to a shallow examination of the problem and an ineffective treatment plan. Without treating the source, the symptoms are likely to return, or the body will adapt in some other way to compensate. You must be prepared not only to advocate for yourself with your doctor, but you need to develop a collaborative relationship. You need someone who will listen, observe, examine you thoroughly, and be open to looking at the bigger picture.

Most doctors have very limited time with patients and they have a huge arsenal of treatments from which to draw—the most handy of which is their prescription pad—so you want to be able to speak intelligently about your symptoms and work with your primary care physician to come up with a treatment plan that will give you the best results—not just a quick fix. Making informed decisions about your health is your right and your responsibility. Don't be afraid to question your doctor, ask for what you need, and keep an open mind about their suggestions. Remember, they work for you and are being paid for their services, but they are not God, and they can't know everything. Approach your medical professionals as if they are your health care team (collaborative health partners) and trust your intuition.

You can treat the symptoms—or you can treat the source. Unfortunately, because of lousy reimbursement and high overhead, physicians are often forced to see patients every ten to fifteen minutes (five minutes of which is spent on documentation). In my experience, it takes more than five to ten minutes with a patient to uncover the clues that help us get to the deeper causes of disease. In that amount of time, they usually only scratch the surface before having to snap to judgment regarding the best plan of care or shuffle you off to a specialist. It's akin to being on a triage team in the battlefield.

The quality of care will be limited by the time the caregiver has to assess the situation, and the tools he has at hand to fix the most immediate problem. You can understand why doctors often take the path of least resistance. Ergo…the physician's script pad. At best, you can hope your doctor is very good at his job, has razor sharp instincts, and is not quick to take that path of least resistance. A good doctor is the one who listens to his patients and trusts that they already know what they need. He will listen for clues and work with you on solutions, rather than dictating what he thinks is best after only a cursory examination. I can't stress how important it is for you to trust your PCP and vice versa.

You are the most important person in your health care team. If I didn't make it clear above, you have choices to make about your health and well-being, and one of the first choices you have is picking your PCP. Choose wisely.

Choosing your PCP

Finding the right doc is a bit like speed dating. You might have to try a few before you find Mr. or Ms. Right, but don't settle on staying with the doctor who gave you your first shot just because he's the family doctor your mother chose forty years ago. I'm not saying there aren't some excellent family doctors who've been in practice for years and have a wealth of knowledge and experience. I'm saying, find the person who is right for you.

Several years ago, when my family doc retired, I was forced to find someone new. I called around to a few doctors' offices within the area I wanted to travel, narrowing my search. Then I researched a dozen or so before whittling it down to five possibilities, all of whom I made sure were covered under my health insurance plan. Of those, I eliminated three with a simple phone call to the office. If I couldn't talk to a real receptionist—preferably one who was helpful and pleasant—within the first three minutes of the call, I hung up. (A nasty receptionist or ten minutes of elevator music is the last thing I want to deal with when I'm sick and trying to reach my doctor.)

When I eliminated all the possibilities on my first choice list, then I widened my search, chose five more, and began again. When I got through to a lovely person on the other end of the phone, I told her who I was and that I was looking for a new PCP. She confirmed that yes, the doctor was taking on new patients. Eureka! Now the real test. I asked these three questions:

1) **How long are appointment times?** This is a straightforward answer that shouldn't take a lot of thought. Office visits should be at least fifteen minutes long and a physical should be thirty. If you're going to the doctor for a chronic problem, it's likely that you have more than one thing going on. Most doctors require separate visits for each issue anyway—their effort to keep the billing and paperwork straight and to avoid patients who come in complaining about everything under the sun. In the case of chronic pain issues, fifteen minutes won't cut it. Especially since wading through all the diagnostic and treatment codes for reimbursement becomes a cumbersome task.

2) **Who will I be seeing when I come in?** Most doctors' offices now have Physician's Assistants (PAs) and Advanced Practice Registered Nurses (APRNs) who routinely see patients in lieu of the physician. This is another way doctors are able to see more patients per day to make up for reduced compensation, cover overhead, and pay the appalling costs of liability insurance. Fortunately, there are some excellent PAs and APRNs in private practices all over the country, pitching in to keep docs afloat and patients seen in a timely manner. I, personally, don't mind seeing them, but if I need to see my doctor, I want to know that I can schedule an appointment directly with him for a serious issue.

3) **And most important to me: How does the doctor feel about Integrative Medicine?** The receptionist might give you some version of, "I don't understand the question," or, "I can't really answer that." This might be one you'll have to reserve for your first office visit, but if the receptionist is quick with a response and says he's for it, he scores big. My favorite doc's exact words were, "If you know of something that works for you, I want to know about it so I can do some research and maybe recommend it to other patients." Bingo! We have

a winner. Humility goes a long way in helping me trust my doctor. I don't expect him to have all the answers and I don't trust anyone who thinks he does. But if I know you're on my team, I'll pretty much follow your lead with confidence, trusting that you have my back and are willing to help me find the right answer.

Once I was in with the doctor, I could tell quickly whether we'd likely hit it off. That may not be important to you. Perhaps you don't feel that your doctor needs to have a great bedside manner. You're only interested in the fact that he's on board with evidence-based integrative medicine and that he'll spend at least fifteen minutes with you when you come in with a problem. That's fine. You don't necessarily want someone who is going to spend the time chatting about their woodworking hobby, but if this new doctor is condescending, dismissive, or otherwise not interested in having a dialogue, I recommend you think twice. You need to have a voice with your doctor. If you don't feel heard, or if the doc isn't getting all the pertinent information to make a proper diagnosis, it won't matter that he's covered under your insurance. He won't likely be able to help you stay well.

If it turns out you've found a compassionate heart and a good listener, as I did, congrats. You've found your man! Or woman. It's important to note here that, like your doctor, you shouldn't snap to judgment after a five minute conversation. If you're a woman, don't jump to the conclusion that you have to have a female doctor or that a woman will be a better listener or more compassionate. I've found equally excellent women doctors as male doctors, and equally arrogant and close minded women as I have men in health care professions. Anyone can have a bad day. Try them out. If you aren't confident that they will give you the level of care you need, find someone else. You aren't marrying them. You're hiring them to work with you. Remember, they are being paid for a service and customer care should be their top priority.

Other concerns to be addressed before your first visit. Check to make sure that your new doctor is indeed covered under your insurance plan. Know your co-payment for office visits and visits to specialists, and find out what hospital your doctor is affiliated with. It might make a difference to you, especially in an emergency situation. If you have an accident, you'll want to know that your doctor has privileges at the hospital you're being taken to. Make sure your medical records are made available to your new doctor so he/she can come up to speed quickly with any pre-existing health issues and ensure that you're caught up on immunizations and tetanus boosters. If you have pertinent X-rays or radiology reports, make sure that the new office has them. Upgraded computerization systems are making this much easier.

Second line of defense

Aside from your PCP (with whom you should consult as needed and see for yearly physicals), you'll want to add members to your team who specialize. Your PCP can probably refer you to a good orthopedist, physical therapist, neurologist, or endocrinologist, but don't just take his word for it. Ask for two or three options so you can decide who the best choice is for you. Investigate. Look them up on Health Grades, an awesome website containing basic facts, patient reviews, and background on listed physicians http://www.healthgrades.com/. Or speak to another health care provider who might have other opinions. The more choices and information you possess, the more control you have regarding your treatment.

Finding Alternative Health Care Providers

Finding a good massage therapist, acupuncturist, chiropractor, or naturopath can be tricky. The best way, in my opinion, is word of mouth. If a trusted friend or other health care provider recommends someone, it's a good bet they've at least had a positive experience with that person. From there, the internet is your friend. Check to see if the proposed practitioner has a website with more information. Also check the professional registries. This will ensure they are in fact licensed, and the registries are great resources for finding providers in your area. Find out if they take your insurance or if you'll be paying out of pocket and how much a session costs.

It needs to be noted here that many alternative health care providers will be an out of pocket expense. Reimbursement for acupuncture and chiropractic care has come a long way, but massage is still considered a "service" industry and is poorly reimbursed, if at all, by insurance companies. But here's how I look at it. I would rather pay $70 an hour for a massage that I know is going to give me lasting benefits and may fix my problem in a few sessions, rather than $40 copays for repeated visits to specialists who only want to give me meds to mask my symptoms or shuffle me off to the next doctor when I don't get better.

You have to be willing to invest in your health, and health maintenance will undoubtedly cost you **time and money…the two main reasons people are generally NOT healthy today.** People want a quick fix, and they want someone else to pay for it. It's simply human nature to look for the easiest solution. Don't take it personally, but this attitude is by far the greatest hindrance to recovery in many cases, especially in situations where people already feel victimized as they often do after car accidents and work related injuries sustained through no fault of their own.

But once a person realizes that a quick fix won't resolve the problem and that blaming others only feeds into negativity, they can come to a new understanding. That taking personal responsibility, becoming invested in your health and wellness, and becoming educated about your choices is the only way to find peace of mind as you navigate the roiling waters of the health care system. Having confidence that you are in control of your body and your health, and that you are in good hands with the team you've chosen will put you on a much faster road to recovery than if you allow yourself to be victimized by a dysfunctional system. Choose consciously and choose wisely.

NOTE: Licensed Massage Therapists should be listed with the AMTA (American Massage Therapy Association). Or you can find local chiropractors, acupuncturists, naturopaths, and osteopaths in your area by checking out www.lifescript.com**. If you're wondering which one you need to see for whatever is ailing you, here's a quick guide that might help you decide, based on what they can do for you.**

Naturopath—A licensed naturopathic physician (ND) is basically your primary care doctor of alternative medicine. An ND attends a four-year, graduate-level naturopathic medical school and is educated in all of the same basic sciences as an MD, but also studies holistic and nontoxic approaches to therapy with a strong emphasis on disease prevention and optimizing wellness. In addition to a standard medical curriculum, the naturopathic physician also studies clinical nutrition, homeopathic medicine, botanical medicine, psychology, and counseling. A naturopathic physician takes rigorous professional board exams so that he or she may be licensed by a state or jurisdiction as a primary care general practice physician. They look at the big picture, may give you advice on nutrition, determine if herbal supplements or homeopathic remedies might be useful, and will be a great resource for finding other alternative healthcare providers.

Osteopath—A DO, Doctor of Osteopathy, can also be a primary care physician. A DO degree is a professional doctoral degree for physicians and surgeons offered by medical schools in the United States. Holders of the DO degree have the ability to become licensed as osteopathic physicians who have equivalent rights, privileges, and responsibilities as physicians with a Doctor of Medicine degree (MD) DO physicians are licensed to practice the full scope of medicine and surgery in 65 countries, including all 50 states in the US, and make up seven percent of the total U.S. physician population. These specialized practitioners look at the whole person and offer skilled hands-on medical procedures that can treat joint malalignments and musculoskeletal disorders. If you think you need to see an orthopedist, but aren't interested in having surgery on whatever ails you, try checking out an Osteopath.

Chiropractor—DC, Doctor of Chiropractic, has a degree from a Chiropractic college but does not have a medical degree. Their main specialty is use of manual manipulation to align the spine. They may use other modalities to treat musculoskeletal injuries, such as electric stim, acupuncture, massage, or therapeutic exercise. A good chiropractor is worth his/her weight in gold. When my back goes really wonky, and I can't fix it myself after a day or two of icing, self-muscle energy techniques, and gentle stretching, I get myself to my chiropractor. Then I schedule a massage and an acupuncture session within the next week. Within 5-7 days, I'm back to yoga and right as rain. Not to mention having a healthy glow to my skin.

Acupuncturist—LAc. requirements are different from state to state but rest assured, Licensed Acupuncturists have had several years of course work and significant clinical practice before they can hang out a shingle. Acupuncture deals with the energetic body. In Traditional Chinese Medicine (TCM), it is believed that the body has natural pathways of energy (meridians), and energy centers (chakras), that can become stagnant or blocked because of injury, illness, poor diet, chronic stress, muscle imbalances, etc. Essentially, our environment and unhealthy lifestyles are conspiring to jam up our chi, and an acupuncturist or TCM practitioner (who may also prescribe Chinese herbal remedies) can help restore the flow and balance of energy in the body. I see acupuncture as a staple in keeping everything flowing optimally and seek treatment on a regular basis. I go seasonally to help me transition and more often when needed for musculoskeletal flare-ups. I also like to combine massage with acupuncture within a few days of each other. My acupuncturist says, "Acupuncture opens the channels and massage moves the fluid and energy along." I like his analogy and would agree with that philosophy wholeheartedly.

NOTE: You have an energy system that needs as much care as your physical, emotional, and spiritual being. Just because you can't see it, or quantify it, doesn't mean it isn't there. Energy medicine has been around for thousands of years across many cultures. Western medicine, by comparison, is still in its infancy at a mere few hundred years of age and limits its focus to biological function rather than holism.

As a practitioner of manual therapy and hands-on treatment, I can tell you that much of what I do is intuitive and done on an energetic level. All of my clients can tell you when I have my hands on them, or even above them, there is heat, there is movement, and yes, most definitely, there is energy. This energy, vital force, electromagnetic current, Qi, Chi, or whatever else you want to call it, effects all of our organ functions and is essential to life and balanced health. Don't ignore it!

Physical Therapist—PTs are your facilitators. They have associates, bachelors, masters and even doctorate level degrees for physical therapy, so know the credentials of who is seeing you. These motivating and skilled professionals are often your first bridge between a Western and Eastern Medicine approach. They look beyond the injury to assess functional return, which often leads to a more holistic approach to care. They can start you on a road to recovery that will include specific exercises, helpful suggestions on body mechanics and practical solutions for quality of life issues. They may also be qualified to do ergonomics assessments and treat overuse injuries. PTs have access to a variety of manual therapy and taping techniques to support proper alignment, and employ the use of ultrasound, electrical stimulation, or even aquatic therapy to aid in the healing process. Continuing education requirements ensure that PTs are at the cutting edge of out-patient rehabilitation.

The greatest drawback is the reduced treatment times in recent years. Thanks to poor reimbursement, endless paperwork, and the high cost of doing business, PT offices are forced—as are other healthcare professionals—to see more patients in less time. No matter how good you are, twenty minutes isn't long enough to give high quality physical therapy care.

Many PT offices today are run like gyms, utilizing physical therapy aides (these are unlicensed but usually trained employees) who will see you through your exercise routine while the PT attends to other patients and checks in with you throughout treatment. Physical therapy aides, physical therapist assistants, and certified athletic trainers (ATCs) are not to be confused. A physical therapist assistant and a certified athletic trainer are licensed health care professionals, usually with an Associate's Degree or a Bachelor's Degree in Exercise Physiology. They are qualified to do most of the same treatments as the physical therapist but are not able to do initial evaluations. Because they have less managerial and administrative duties, however, they sometimes have more one on one time with patients, which can be a bonus.

Massage Therapists—LMTs, as in every profession, are not all created equal. Some may have gone through an intensive training program over a two or three year period, while others have become certified in less than a year. Each state has its own regulations regarding how many hours of training constitutes eligibility for licensure. For some, it's 500, and others, it's 750 hours. You might also want to understand that while some massage programs lean toward spa massage, others may focus on medical massage. Either way, they may have a good understanding of anatomy and physiology and have excellent massage technique, but lack the experience of working within a medical profession. It's not to say you won't get good care and a great massage, but if you need spinal adjustment, you usually would seek out an osteopath, chiropractor, or physical therapist who does muscle energy work or practices manual therapy.

There are many specialties within the realm of hands-on therapies, from Reiki to cranio-sacral therapy and myofascial release to Thai massage. I offer all of these services in my practice but specialize in deep tissue massage and neuromuscular facilitation, or muscle energy techniques, which are used to correct spinal alignment and restore muscle balance. I had the great privilege of training with some of the best physical therapists in the Northeast, and over a period of twenty years in the orthopedic outpatient and sports medicine field, I honed my skills as a manual therapist. That's the kind of extra something you want from your providers. Exceptional practitioners may be few and far between, but they're out there. It's up to you to find them.

CHAPTER 5

FIGHTING THE BATTLE OF THE BULGE

With your health in the hands of a trusted team, now is the time for you to take action. The first order of business is facing the proverbial elephant in the room. Have you been avoiding mirrors, wearing nothing but "stretchy" clothes, and reveling in the "live large and enjoy life" philosophy with gusto? If your health is excellent, you could care less what the scale—or Aunt Josephine—has to say, and you are happy just as you are, feel free to skip this section. But if you're like most people—even when you're smiling on the outside—if you aren't in your best shape, you don't feel well or satisfied with yourself. And here's some news for you ladies, men have the same self-image issues that we do. They may or may not talk about it, but they struggle with the same feeling of helplessness about their weight as women do. Whoever you are, if you're ready to educate yourself and make a commitment to improving your life, read on.

Before we go any further, I'd like to reframe the word "weight-loss" and instead, refer to the subject as "weight management." This takes the focus off the problem as a short term goal to lose weight and makes it more of a lifestyle choice that will become part of your daily routine. Just like oral hygiene or skin care, you can approach weight management as an ongoing daily practice. Thinking of it this way takes the burden off of being perfect with every choice you make. You may try to brush your teeth three times a day and floss twice, but more than likely, it's a two out of three success. You don't beat yourself up for forgetting to floss. You just do it the next day and give it your best effort to stay on track so when you visit the dentist, you don't have to pay for your laxity with cavities and expensive dental work.

If you can **consider your eating habits as part of your weight management plan**, you'll do your best to make good choices daily. You'll plan your meals, watch your portion sizes, and choose carefully how you want to "spend" your daily allowance of calories. Moderation in all things is key, but allowing yourself some "wiggle" room will make you a happier and healthier person. I go by the 80/20 rule. If I eat right and get enough exercise 80% of the time, I can ease up, take a day off, and eat what I want 20% of the time. But that also means that I'm not going to be a "perfect" size "4"…or "6," or "8," depending on your version of what's ideal. I'm okay with that and you have to learn to be too if you don't want to keep feeling like a failure every time you step out of line.

One of the pitfalls of being on a "diet" is the restrictive nature of it. It feels punitive and induces guilt when we stray. These are not positive re-enforcements by any means and will likely sabotage your efforts. I recall an old Garfield cartoon that showed the orange tabby with a miserable look on his face, and a caption that read, "I tried a diet once. It was the worst fifteen minutes of my life." I don't know about you, but as soon as I say the word "diet," I want to eat everything I shouldn't. It's just the way we rebellious humans are wired.

A more effective approach is to keep in mind all the foods you CAN eat. We generally shop from the same list of about twenty-five to thirty items. Check out your favorite healthy meals and create an ingredients list with thirty to forty "diet approved" foods, and shop only from that list. Know where these items are in the store and make a bee-line for them when you hit the grocery store. Don't be sidetracked by the snack, soda, or bread aisle and watch out for those end cap traps. You know the shelves at the end of each aisle that have three bags of chips for the price of two, or twelve cans of gravy for a dollar. **Resist buying unhealthy foods simply because they're cheap.**

Weigh in weekly—NOT daily. "Chronic dieters" hate the scale. They see it as the enemy and either avoid it altogether, or force themselves onto it daily only to have their hopes dashed when they don't see the results of having sacrificed that third slice of pizza the night before. Weight can fluctuate on a daily basis by as much as five pounds, depending on what you've eaten, how much water you're retaining, and whatever hormonal upheaval is happening in your body. Weighing in daily can be discouraging and counterproductive. However, avoiding the scale altogether is a bad idea. It's much easier to catch yourself when you only have to take off five or ten pounds than it is to wait until you've gained an entire pants size in the month since you last weighed in. Try not to obsess about the numbers, but be willing to face the cold hard truth head on so you can do something about it. Just because you aren't looking at a problem doesn't mean it isn't there. Use the numbers to motivate you. Celebrate your successes—not with food rewards please—and brush off the "failures" as lessons learned about what you need to be doing differently.

On that note, I want to add, embrace who you are. If being overweight truly doesn't bother you and you're living a full, happy life, then embrace it. Wear your "bigness" with pride and don't let anyone make you feel bad about it. But if your health is suffering and you're constantly battling with feelings of low self-esteem because of your weight, do something about it. **Feeling guilty and hating yourself serves no one and will undoubtedly keep you stuck in your rut.**

As much as I'd love to say the solution to obesity is simply to "move more, eat less," there is nothing simple about the overweight and obesity epidemic in this country. **For adults,** overweight and obesity ranges are measured by using weight and height to compute the person's BMI (Body Mass Index). The BMI is used because, for most people, it correlates with the amount of fat in their bodies. I'll talk about this more in a few minutes.

These statistics are a bit on the old side now, and data collection/compilation/publishing is always a few years behind, but the following statistics are telling nonetheless. Data from the National Health and Nutrition Examination Survey, 2009–2010 shows:

- More than 2 in 3 adults are considered to be overweight or obese.
- More than 1 in 3 adults are considered to be obese.
- More than 1 in 20 adults are considered to have extreme obesity.
- About one-third of children and adolescents ages 6 to 19 are considered to be overweight or obese.
- More than 1 in 6 children and adolescents ages 6 to 19 are considered to be obese

NOTE: Children grow at different rates at different times, so it's not always easy to tell if a child is overweight. BMI charts for children compare their height and weight to other children of their same sex and age, but we need to consider body type and growth spurts as factors as well. A child may appear to be overweight due to a widening and spreading out that precedes a period of rapid growth. We don't want to inadvertently contribute to negative body images in children by putting them on a "diet" because they are a bit on the pudgy side at the age of eight or have a "husky" build when they hit their pre-pubescent eleventh year and are eating us out of house and home. The best advice for

parents of these kids is to set a good example, offer healthy choices, and keep kids active through sports and every day play.

The issue of being overweight or obese is a multifaceted problem requiring a multi-disciplinary approach.

On the whole, here are what I see as the major contributing factors to the overweight/obesity epidemic:

- **Decreased physical activity** due to technological demands and lifestyle/societal changes.
- **Reduced quality of food sources.** The majority of our foods are overly processed, loaded with sugar and chemicals, and are grown from over-farmed, nutrient deficient soil.
- **The Marketing machine** that drives us to spend our hard earned dollar on a two liter bottle of soda or a .99 cent Big Gulp rather than a half-gallon container of organic milk that costs four times as much, is at the core of malnutrition problems in an obese society. It's hard to imagine, but most people who are overweight are actually malnourished. When the body is not receiving proper nutrients, it goes into starvation mode. Without balanced, healthy nutrition, it becomes almost impossible to escape the primal, physiologic desire for carbs and fats to sustain us. This problem is exacerbated by abundantly available, cheap and easy carbs, and unhealthy fats that are cleverly and insidiously marketed to consumers. We are bombarded at every turn with advertisements to buy more of what is bad for us. When was the last time you saw a commercial touting the healthy deliciousness of fresh fruits and vegetables and the importance of buying organic? No doubt, you'll notice most food commercials represent fast food restaurants and highly processed foods. In other words, the cards are stacked against us making healthy choices.
- **Rampant rise in cases of Metabolic Syndrome** (I'll explain what this is in detail shortly). Research shows an increase in Metabolic Syndrome in American adults from 29 % in surveys done between 1988-1994, to 34% in a similar study done between 2000 and 2006. In general, the researchers found the rise in metabolic syndrome was primarily due to growing rates of abdominal obesity and high blood pressure. Today's numbers are likely staggering in comparison.
- **Fast paced, high stress lifestyles** cause a rise in cortisol and other "weight gain" hormones, leading to adrenal fatigue, high blood pressure, and a myriad of other health problems, all contributing to weight gain. **I'll address this later in the section on STRESS MANAGEMENT.**
- **Sleep deprivation** inhibits the body's recovery and interferes with hormonal balance, contributing to the Metabolic Syndrome I mentioned above. According to News Max Health, in its first International Bedroom Poll, the National Sleep Foundation determined citizens of the United States and Japan between the ages of 25 and 55 get less sleep—on average—than four other nations: Canada, Mexico, the United Kingdom, and Germany. More than half of Americans surveyed say they sleep less than seven hours on work nights, compared to two-thirds of Japanese, 39 percent of Brits, 36 percent of Germans, 30 percent of Canadians, and 29 percent of Mexicans. Americans are working more and sleeping less—and growing fatter.
- **Social pressures and body image** are huge factors in weight management. We live in a society that values thinness (according to every magazine cover, television show, or movie you see), yet we are a culture that super-sizes every meal. Portion sizes in America are three to five times larger than the normal recommended, so we are now conditioned to eat more, yet expected to weigh less. That's a tough dichotomy to live with. And an impossible expectation to achieve. In addition, since most of us

equate social gatherings with an abundance of food, alcohol, and sweets, we are inundated with poor choices, large portions, and positive reinforcement in the form of emotional connection to others around food.

- **Emotional connection.** Food, for many of us, triggers complicated emotional messages with powerful connections to childhood and security. The serotonin boost we get from sugars and fats mimic the same chemical responses we get from emotions such as love, acceptance, and feeling nurtured and secure. There are almost always issues of control, reward, and punishment around food and eating, going back to a time before you can even remember your first "snack food" or "treat."

The emotional component is by far the hardest piece of the puzzle to solve, and often requires significant counseling and retraining the mind—a terrifying and daunting proposition for most people. No one wants to dredge up the past, delve into their dysfunctional childhood, or relive those times when your mom, worried about you not eating enough, forced you to sit at the table until you ate all your peas. More people have developed a hate for green vegetables this way than I can possibly count. Not to mention attaching guilt to food by insisting you consider the starving children in Africa who would die for those peas. They reward you with "sweets" and unwittingly attach punishment to "healthy" foods.

Moms and Dads aren't trying to scar you for life. They are trying to teach you to appreciate what you have, eat a variety of foods, and get enough healthy nutrition so you can grow big and strong. But despite their good intentions, somewhere along the line, nutrition becomes a control issue and the messages get jumbled in our psyches, leading us to a lifetime of bad eating habits, guilt, and lack of control around food—especially if parents are dealing with their own issues around food. Unlearning those old messages is tough enough, but replacing them with new ways of thinking and relating to food requires time, effort, and commitment—not to mention, discipline.

Yup, I said the "D" word. Discipline has such a negative connotation to it. We immediately think of punishment. Self-discipline is even nastier. Now, I'm expected to dole out punishment upon myself. Depriving myself of foods I love and punishing myself with guilt over being "weak" are two of the biggest enemies of weight management.

After watching a few seasons of *The Biggest Loser*, it became clear to me that success or failure of a contestant to lose weight, and later for them to keep the weight off, was more about them dealing with their "demons" than anything else they got out of being on the show.

In an atmosphere where food is prepared, healthy choices are consistently provided, and intense daily training is a requirement, folks are bound to see significant weight loss. But once they get out into the real world, if they haven't dealt with the reasons why they overeat, and why they make the choices they do about their lifestyles, the success will be short lived. One of the things I love about that show is that the trainers get that. They push the contestants hard physically, but they also push them to deal with their emotional and psychological hurdles. They give them the education to make the best choices, and then they root out the underlying causes to their obesity.

This type of retraining is called Cognitive Behavioral Therapy (CBT). The underlying concept behind CBT is that our thoughts and feelings play a fundamental role in our behavior. For example, a person who spends a lot of time thinking about plane crashes, runway accidents, and other air disasters may find themselves avoiding air travel. The goal of cognitive behavioral therapy is to teach patients that while they cannot control every aspect of the world around them, they can take control of how they interpret and deal with things in their environment.

Gandhi once said:
"Keep your thoughts positive because your thoughts become your words.
Keep your words positive because your words become your behaviors.
Keep your behaviors positive because your behaviors become your habits.
Keep your habits positive because your habits become your values.
Keep your values positive because your values become your destiny."

The short version of this sentiment is that thoughts lead to feelings, feelings lead to actions, and actions lead to consequences (results). What this boils down to for our weight management goals is that the battle of the bulge is won in the mind.

Cognitive behavioral therapy has become increasingly popular in recent years with both mental health consumers and treatment professionals. Because CBT is usually a short-term treatment option, it is often more affordable than some other types of therapy. CBT is also empirically supported and has been shown to effectively help patients overcome a wide variety of maladaptive behaviors.

I'll leave it to you, Gandhi, and a psychotherapist to fix your emotional and spiritual problems, but now that you know your issues around food aren't going anywhere until you decide to do something about them, you can stop sweeping them under the rug and recognize the need for real change. For now, let's at least deal with some of these other issues. In the following section, I'll give some practical solutions to the problems I mentioned above regarding the factors contributing to obesity.

We can definitely do something about our **decreased activity level**. I've already offered some suggestions earlier in the book but here are a few reminders:

- **Drink plenty of water.** I know I'm repeating myself, but not only will hydration keep your body working optimally, reduce your tendency to snack, and give your skin a healthy glow, **it will also force you to get up frequently** to hit the bathroom. While you're up, you can do a few of the stretches I'll give you later in the book.
- **Try a treadmill desk, fit desk, or standing desk. Take frequent stretch breaks and add mini workouts to your work day.**
- **Make fitness a family affair.** Set a good example for your children to show them you value fitness. Include them in your workouts (kids love Zumba and yoga), and find family friendly activities you can do together. Skiing, ice skating, hiking, biking, camping, and swimming are just a few ideas for ways to spend family time in motion. I spent a lot of time roller blading with my youngest and was a team mom for all of my kids' sports. We did Boy Scouts together (being a Scout leader for fifteen years was one of the best times of my life), and even now, I take my granddaughter to a weekly tumble and splash

class at the local YMCA. Exercising together encourages communication, emphasizes shared goals, and offers an outlet for stress relief. You'll never regret the moments you spend with your kids. Share your love for fitness—a tremendous gift that will keep giving throughout their lives. Also important to note is that spouses who work out together often have a deeper connection and can better support each other when it comes to making healthy choices about diet and nutrition.

- **Schedule exercise time. There is NO excuse not to exercise. Stop trying to find one.**
- **Limit screen time for you and your family. Initiate a "tech-fast" day a few times per month where NO devices are used for a full day. Don't treat it like a punishment. Instead, take the family on a day trip to a museum, see a live show or concert, or try a whole weekend of camping and leave the gadgets at home. Play games, be active, and talk instead. You'll be amazed at what conversations are brought about.**

I'll take the next two problems together. Finding high quality food sources and avoiding the "buy me" trap of the "Marketing machine."

"You are what you eat."
This statement has never been truer. Finding high quality, nutrient dense foods is challenging at best. Finding them at affordable prices makes the search even more difficult. But with some effort and creative financing, it can be done. As I mentioned above, our soil is depleted and many of our food sources have been highly processed or loaded with chemicals and pesticides or have been genetically modified in some way. The jury is still out on the long term effects of GMOs, but my gut—and recent research—tells me it's not a good thing. Look it up. Read the literature, and decide for yourself.

The food industry is a complex web of producers, distributors, and consumers. Without farms and farmers, we would have no food. They are the producers. All over the world, farmers grow food, raise livestock, and manage crops so that seven billion people may remain fed daily. It's an enormous task, but somehow we have managed to create and keep in place, a viable system for feeding the masses. But despite our ability to grow an abundance of food in some parts of the world, others starve. The problem in this case is not the lack of food but a break down in distribution channels. Whether corporate greed or political sabotage and social decay are at fault is a discussion for another book, but suffice it to say, it's complicated.

On the consumer end of the process, we are like lambs to the slaughter. The science of marketing is a multi-billion dollar industry in itself. Food manufacturers have a captive audience since we all need to eat, but competition is fierce for that shelf-space in the grocery store, so they have to make their products stand out. Trust me, they have done their homework and know what sells, why it sells, and who they can sell it to. They have made it their mission to ensure that we become "addicted" to their products and will keep coming back for more. This is why most processed foods are loaded with sugar, salt, and chemical additives that not only provide a longer shelf life but that appeal to our taste buds. There's even a science to packaging products that sell. It's all very subliminal and creepy in my opinion, but you get the picture.

Don't be a drone. Look past the pretty packaging and read the fine print. Know what you're spending your hard earned dollars on and get the highest quality product for the best price. It takes practice to see past the BS, but if you're mindful about your purchases, you'll get a feel for what's worth the extra money and what's not. Fast, easy, and cheap doesn't translate to quality food in our society, so don't be sucked into the trap of thinking, "it's too hard and expensive to eat healthy." This is a lie! If you take some time to educate yourself about what's healthy and what's not, and take time to shop smart, I can guarantee you'll come to realize that buying and preparing healthy meals for you and your family will SAVE you money in the long run. Eating nutrient dense, healthy foods will keep you more satisfied, help you EAT LESS, and will ultimately save you on health care costs down the road. Keep track of how often you're eating out and what you spend on snacks you pick up on the fly, and compare that to what it would cost you to pack healthy snacks and lunches from home. Trust me, you'll be shocked at the cost savings.

I've had to become somewhat obsessive about choices I make at the grocery store. I choose organic fruits and vegetables whenever possible, shop at stores that carry a good selection of whole foods, and seasonally seek out local organic farmers. I understand that not all foods labeled "organic" are "guaranteed" but certainly my chances are better at getting higher quality, fresh foods from nearby farmers. Check into your local food co-ops, often run by health food stores and farmer's' markets. You can get an incredible amount of wholesome food for a reasonable price when you buy in bulk. At the same time, you'll be supporting a local business and avoiding the sharks. Learn to freeze or can extras or use them in smoothies. Make it a point to know where health food stores, farm-to-table restaurants, and organic juice bars within driving distance are, so when you cruise past those fast food joints at lunch time, you have a destination to go where you'll have consistently healthy choices that you can trust.

Not that there aren't some good options at most restaurants these days, but when faced with ordering an egg white veggie omelet or a Boston cream doughnut at the corner DD, umm…I'm just not that strong. And have you tasted how salty those egg white omelets are? Aside from wanting to avoid temptation, I want to know, as much as is possible, where my food comes from and how it's prepared. If I can't see an ingredients list, I don't know what I'm getting. There are only a few juice bar/health food type restaurants within twenty-five miles of me, but any one of them is worth the drive to find delicious, nutritious meals that I can tailor to my needs. In a pinch, I visit the local deli or salad bar at the grocery store and choose things like kale or edamame salad, add a protein rich scoop of tuna or cottage cheese and stick to the olive oil and vinegar for dressing.

Negotiating the gauntlet that is our local grocery store is a challenge. Learn to become a label reader. Understand what is in your food and what you are feeding your body. At the very least, familiarize yourself with common ingredients to avoid. If you see the words, high fructose corn syrup (HFCS), hydrogenated oils, soy (most of which has been genetically modified), or lists of chemicals, colors, flavors, and dyes you can't pronounce, consider skipping that item and replacing it with something less processed.

Read the labels and understand the food you're buying.

I'm not suggesting that you become obsessed with food, count every calorie, or become a food Nazi at parties. I'm only suggesting that you be mindful of how you're fueling your body, and commit to educating yourself so that the choices you make are informed and conscious.

Include chicken, fish, and beans into your meal makeover.

Chicken, fish, and beans are loaded with protein and have less saturated fat than beef, pork, and lamb. These food winners have been shown to improve heart health, brain function, and digestion. Organic chicken is best and should be eaten sans skin, and baked, broiled, grilled, or poached—never breaded or fried. Beans are loaded with fiber, giving them the added benefit of making you feel fuller, but avoid canned beans with added syrups and preservatives. If you don't have time to soak and cook your own (pressure cookers make this relatively quick and easy), go for the organic canned beans and rinse them before adding them to your meal. The old baked beans with molasses and added sugar are not recommended…sorry franks and beans lovers! Try adding a variety of beans to soups, stews, and salads. Lentils, chick peas, navy beans, and cannellini beans for instance, add an awesome extra taste and texture to any meal.

To fish or not to fish? According to most health sources, you should plan at least two fish meals per week, one being that of an oily fish such as salmon, sardines, or tuna. Fish are loaded with lean protein and essential vitamins and minerals. Oily fish in particular has heart-healthy omega-3 fatty acids, including DHA, the fatty acid that nourishes the brain.

NOTE: To avoid mercury and toxins, exclude sword fish, shark, tilefish, and king mackerel altogether. Limit tuna consumption to no more than six ounces per week, and limit shellfish consumption like clams, oysters, lobster, and scallops which feed on industrial deposits, sewage, and the waste of other fish, filtering it through their own bodies. I, personally, love these little "hoovers" of the ocean but do try to eat them only once or twice a month at most. Stick to wild caught salmon rather than farm raised, which have higher fat content and may contain preservatives, dyes, and antibiotics.

Fish should be baked, steamed, poached, or grilled. Avoid deep fat frying!

CAUTION: Pregnant and breast-feeding women, children, and babies should limit intake of seafood, fish, and shellfish. Please consult your doctor or health care professional for more advice on this. NRDC (Natural Resources Defense Council) has a great guide on their website to help you make informed choices about your fish and seafood consumption. http://www.nrdc.org/oceans/seafoodguide/

Support sustainable fishing practices by buying certified sustainable or by going to Conservation Alliance for Seafood Solutions for more information at http://www.solutionsforseafood.org

Variety is the Spice of Life

Incorporating a wide variety of colorful fruits and veggies into your diet is essential to keeping you healthy and functioning at your optimal best. There are so many healthy and incredible tasting fruits and vegetables that there is NO EXCUSE not to be eating them on a daily basis. The recommended two to four servings of fruits and three to five servings of veggies per day may seem like a lot, but there are awesome ways to fit these powerhouses of nutrition into your day. Organic vegetable juices and smoothies are one way to easily meet the requirements (See the section on **PJ's Favorite Smoothie Recipes**).

Adding a variety of vegetables and fruits to salads is another. My salads are "famous" with my friends and family for being packed with flavor and nutrition. I almost always add fruit in the form of chopped apples, pears, grapes, or melon, along with nuts, seeds, olives, and avocado to balance it out with some healthy fats. **Be careful of these additions if you're trying to lose weight, and add only one or two "sweet" or "healthy fat" ingredients since they are high in calories.**

As for veggies, think in terms of a rainbow of color. Brightly colored foods like peppers, squashes, and carrots are delicious and nutritious as well as bringing a splash of beauty to any plate, meal, or salad. And don't forget your green leafy veggies—to be eaten at least three times per week. Spinach, kale, chard, and cruciferous vegetables like broccoli and cauliflower are loaded with essential vitamins and minerals. You can't go wrong with stocking your fridge with fresh, organic produce to give your family lots of options for snacking as well as mealtimes. If you haven't gotten to them within a few days, they make for excellent juicing/smoothie ingredients.

NOTE ON BUYING ORGANIC: Do try to buy organic fruits and vegetables whenever possible but realize they won't keep as long as non-organic produce so you may have to shop more frequently.

The following information was published in 2010 on PBS.org.

A report issued by the President's Cancer Panel recommends eating produce without pesticides to reduce your risk of getting cancer and other diseases. And according to the Environmental Working Group (an organization of scientists, researchers, and policymakers), certain types of organic produce can reduce the amount of toxins you consume on a daily basis by as much as 80 percent.

The group put together two lists, "The Dirty Dozen" and "The Clean 15," to help consumers know when they should buy organic and when it is unnecessary. These lists were compiled using data from the United States Department of Agriculture on the amount of pesticide residue found in non-organic fruits and vegetables *after* they had been washed.

The fruits and vegetables on "The Dirty Dozen" list, when conventionally grown, tested positive for at least 47 different chemicals, with some testing positive for as many as 67. For produce on the "dirty" list, you should definitely go organic—unless you relish the idea of consuming a chemical cocktail. "The Dirty Dozen" list includes:

- celery
- peaches
- strawberries
- apples
- domestic blueberries
- nectarines
- sweet bell peppers
- spinach, kale, and collard greens
- cherries
- potatoes

- imported grapes

- lettuce

All the produce on "The Clean 15" bore little to no traces of pesticides and are safe to consume in non-organic form. This list includes:

- onions

- avocados

- sweet corn

- pineapples

- mango

- sweet peas

- asparagus

- kiwi fruit

- cabbage

- eggplant

- cantaloupe

- watermelon

- grapefruit

- sweet potatoes

- sweet onions

Why are some types of produce more prone to sucking up pesticides than others? Richard Wiles, senior vice president of policy for the Environmental Working Group says, "If you eat something like a pineapple or sweet corn, they have a protection defense because of the outer layer of skin. Not the same for strawberries and berries, which are porous."

The President's Cancer Panel recommends washing conventionally grown produce to remove residues. Wiles adds, "You should do what you can do, but the idea you are going to wash pesticides off is a fantasy. But you should still wash it because you will reduce pesticide exposure."

Remember, the lists of dirty and clean produce were compiled after the USDA washed the produce using high-power pressure water systems that many of us could only dream of having in our kitchens.

The full list contains 49 types of produce, rated on a scale of least to most pesticide residue. You can check out the full list on the Environmental Working Group's website at www.foodnews.org.

I hope I've given you the tools to set you on the road to becoming your best self—the person you were meant to be. Now that you know the numbers you need to focus on, you can set some clear goals and make the necessary adjustments to your diet and exercise life. Write out that healthy grocery list, clear out the junk food, and start today. Take a long walk. You have nothing to lose…except for a few pounds.

CHAPTER 6

METABOLIC SYNDROME
(AND WHY "DIETS" DON'T WORK)

Metabolic syndrome is not a disease in itself. Instead, it's a group of risk factors—including **high blood pressure** (135/80 or higher), **high blood sugar** (100 mg/dl or higher), **unhealthy cholesterol levels** (high triglycerides of 150 mg/dl and/or low HDL of less than 40 mg/dl for men and less than 50 mg/dl for women), **and abdominal fat** (40+ inch waist measurement for men, or 35+ inches for women). To be diagnosed with Metabolic Syndrome, you must have at least three of these conditions. According to the American Heart Association, a staggering 47 million Americans have it. That's one out of every six people!

Any one of these conditions is cause for concern, but with each contributing risk factor your chances for stroke, heart attack, and Type 2 Diabetes grows exponentially. But here's the good news. Metabolic syndrome can be completely reversed by addressing—and reversing—each of these conditions with proper nutrition and exercise. The problem is, that if you have all, or even some of these conditions, your metabolism has slowed to a snail's pace and it can be extremely difficult to get it going again. So here's the deal.

The first thing you need to do is become educated about what contributes to a slow metabolism. **One of the main culprits is hormonal imbalance.** The fat storing hormone, T3 (made by your thyroid) goes into overdrive when you are suddenly trying to limit calories or binge diet. At the same time, Ghrelin (the hunger hormone that entices you to choose chocolate cake over leafy greens) is produced in higher quantities, and Leptin (the hormone that inhibits hunger in order to regulate energy balance and fat storage), is nearly shut off completely. There is significant evidence that we are genetically predisposed to how these hormones work in our body and how receptive they are to stimuli. Thanks Mom and Dad. It seems a cruel irony, but it's also your body's way of keeping you from starving during a famine.

So how do we overcome this terrible plight, you ask? The simple answer is that we eat more! You heard me correctly. I'm also certain I'm not the first person you've heard say this if you've been around the diet circuit. The trick to losing weight is about maintaining hormone balance, blood sugar levels, and calorie input/output. In a nutshell, you need to keep your body fueled throughout the day to keep your endocrine system working optimally and avoid the blood sugar highs and lows.

What you need to know about yourself to make this work is how many calories you actually need to consume to maintain or lose weight. Let's first find our BMR (Basal Metabolic Rate), not to be confused with BMI (Body Mass Index), which I'll get to in a moment. BMR is the measurement used to determine how many calories a day your body needs to maintain basic functions.

NOTE: Realize that a person with very lean muscle mass will burn more calories and a person with a high percentage of body fat will burn less. There are BMR calculators online to help you figure out your number, but if you're a math whiz and want to tackle the numbers on your own, here are the

standard formulas:

English BMR Formula

Women: BMR = 655 + (4.35 x weight in pounds) + (4.7 x height in inches) - (4.7 x age in years)
Men: BMR = 66 + (6.23 x weight in pounds) + (12.7 x height in inches) - (6.8 x age in years)

Metric BMR Formula

Women: BMR = 655 + (9.6 x weight in kilos) + (1.8 x height in cm) - (4.7 x age in years)
Men: BMR = 66 + (13.7 x weight in kilos) + (5 x height in cm) - (6.8 x age in years)

For example, if you are a 40 year old American woman who weighs 160 pounds and is 5'3" (we'll call her Mary Jane), your calculation would look like this:

655 + (4.35 x 160) + (4.7 x 63) – 40 = 1460

NOTE: This is the calories needed for basic function of your organ systems and survival. It is NOT recommended that you decrease your daily calorie intake below this number for an extended period of time as your body will begin cannibalizing muscle tissue and you risk damage to organ systems with prolonged caloric deficits. This is often what happens to people with eating disorders such as anorexia and bulimia, who either severely restrict calories or binge and then purge. If you or someone you know suffers from an eating disorder, there is help. http://www.nationaleatingdisorders.org/

Now that you know your BMR, determine your total daily calorie needs by multiplying your BMR by the appropriate activity factor, as follows:

If you are:

Sedentary (little or no exercise): multiply BMR x 1.2
Lightly active (light exercise/sports 1-3 days/week): multiply BMR x 1.375
Moderately active (moderate exercise/sports 3-5 days/week): multiply BMR x 1.55
Very active (hard exercise/sports 6-7 days a week): Multiply BMR x 1.725
Extra active (very hard exercise/sports & physical job, or 2x/day training): multiply BMR x 1.9

This will give you the number of calories per day you need to maintain your current weight. From here it isn't difficult to determine how many calories per day you need to add or subtract to increase or decrease your weight.

Let's refer to our example of Mary Jane, the 40-year-old woman with a BMR of 1460 (rounded up from 1459). If she has a desk job and only gets out for walks three days a week and doesn't do much more than that, we would consider her to be **sedentary**, multiply her BMR x 1.2, and calculate that she needs approximately 1752 calories per day to maintain her current weight of 160 pounds.

Here is where BMI comes in. Body Mass Index is the standard measurement today's health care professionals use to determine healthy weight. It takes into consideration a person's height/weight ratio and a person's age. There are charts for both men and women available online, as well as BMI calculators so you can see where you stand. As you may have gathered, I'm not an absolutist. I use numbers as guidelines but recognize that they often don't take into account important factors. Genetics play a role in body type and some people inherently have more lean muscle mass, making their height/weight ratio a bit less cut and dried.

Underweight = <18.5
Normal weight = 18.5–24.9
Overweight = 25–29.9
Obesity = BMI of 30 or greater

According to the BMI calculator, our test subject, Mary Jane, has a BMI of between 28 and 29. She is on the upper end of the overweight scale bordering on obese. Clearly, an 1800+ calorie a day diet is doing her no favors, but if she is an active person who works out five days a week, exhibits good cardiovascular endurance, and has a balanced healthy diet, she probably can carry her 160 pounds pretty well and still be healthy. Will she feel even better at twenty pounds lighter and have a better self-image? Probably. This is a quality of life issue. If she is comfortable in her skin, wears her size 10/12 with pride, and has no limitations in her activities of daily living, kudos. Enjoy that extra glass of wine and second helping of mashed potatoes and keep on truckin', sister! But over time, realize that this behavior will likely take its toll in high cholesterol, heart disease, or increased risk of stroke and cancer.

Another helpful (if not depressing) measurement to consider is waist circumference. Measuring waist circumference helps screen for possible health risks that come with being overweight and assessing obesity. If most of your fat is around your waist rather than at your hips, you're at a higher risk for heart disease and type 2 Diabetes. This risk goes up with a waist size that is greater than 35 inches for women or greater than 40 inches for men. To correctly measure your waist, stand and place a tape measure around your middle, just above your hipbones. Measure your waist just after you breathe out.

> **If that number looks suspect, don't freak out! Instead, choose to do something about it. If you recognize the need to lose a few pounds, here's what to do next.**

Considering a pound of fat is equal to 3500 calories, in order to lose a pound of fat per week (we don't want to lose lean muscle mass), you'll need to either reduce your calorie intake by 500 calories per day, or burn 500 more calories per day. If you've ever been on a piece of exercise equipment and slaved to burn even 250 calories in an hour, you know that it's daunting to try to burn an extra 500 calories in a day. And asking our friend Mary Jane to shrink her diet to a mere 1250 calories per day would simply be torture. So, to set Mary Jane up for success, I would recommend that she reduce her daily calories by 250 and increase her daily calorie expenditure by 250. This allows her a healthy 1500 calories/day diet and requires her to kick up her activity level to burn that extra 250 calories/day. It's a very doable solution!

These are my best suggestions for conquering a sluggish metabolism.

- **Eat small, frequent meals.** If you've determined that you need 1500 calories a day to lose a pound a week, break up your meal plan as follows.

250 calorie breakfast:
Suggestions include, an egg, a piece of whole grain toast, and a quarter cup of cottage cheese. Or a cup of plain Greek yogurt with slivered almonds, cinnamon, and a few drops of vanilla extract. For a quick grab-and-go breakfast, I like to prepare a batch of steel cut oatmeal on Sunday mornings. I cook it in almond/coconut milk, divide it into half cup serving sized containers, and reheat them as needed throughout the week, adding some walnuts, fruit, and cinnamon for a yummy, satisfying breakfast.

150 calorie mid-morning snack: (high fiber and/or high protein).
A handful of almonds, an apple with almond butter, or a yogurt.

300-400 calorie lunch:
This could be a salad (watch out for highly processed, high fat/high sugar dressings). Soups and sandwiches are also an option, but think about the quality of the ingredients. Are there additives and preservatives? Canned soups with high sodium content and breads made with HFCS (high fructose corn syrup) are to be avoided, so KNOW where your food is coming from. It's best to pack lunches at home so you can control your serving sizes and know exactly what you're eating. A nutrient dense smoothie is another excellent choice for lunch.

100-150 calorie afternoon snack:
A hardboiled egg is only about sixty calories. Or if you're looking for something sweet, have a piece of fruit, a handful of dark chocolate covered almonds, or even a Weight Watchers ice cream sandwich. Depriving yourself will only make you want to binge.

6-700 calorie dinner:
Baked, poached, or broiled chicken, fish, or lean organic meats. Add a heaping serving of your favorite veggies and a small portion of whole grains (brown rice, quinoa, or whole grain bread). Add something calcium rich to your meal like cottage cheese, leafy greens, or coconut milk (I use it for cooking my rice), and you'll satisfy your cravings as well as helping adjust your fat-burning machinery.

Close the kitchen after dinner

Consider the kitchen closed after you've cleaned up the dinner dishes. Turn out the light, put a lock on the freezer door (or whatever it takes to keep **everyone** out), and set a good example for kids by eliminating the after 7 p.m. sweets and snacks.

This model works! Because you are eating frequently, your blood sugar will remain steady, Ghrelin levels will decrease, and leptin levels will rise, making you feel satisfied, reducing your cravings for sweets, and curbing your urge to binge. If you know you're going out for dinner, set in your mind ahead of time how many calories you can have at dinner to keep with your calorie input/output plan, and modify your intake throughout the day to accommodate for what will likely be a 1000 calorie meal or more. A Bloomin' Onion at Outback is 1500 calories, so choose wisely when the menu comes. And don't forget to count alcohol. It's easy to derail your best intentions when you're hungry and everything looks good…especially if you are plying your self-control with a second glass of wine (@~130 calories per glass)! Is it any wonder why waiters take our drink order first?

- **Add plyometric (jump training) to your workouts.** Jump training boosts metabolism like crazy. It also has the side benefit of increasing bone density and improving muscular endurance, balance, and agility. Obviously, if you have ankle, hip, knee, or spine/disc problems, you'll have to consider alternatives (try jumping on a mini trampoline for less impact, or do water aerobics instead of dry-land jump training). Having said that, if you're healthy and generally fit, don't be afraid to try it. Speed rope, jumping jacks, or even jogging in place are doable for most people. Start slow, test the waters, and then jump in!
- **Interval training.** Our bodies adapt quickly to exercise. Although daily walking on the treadmill is of some benefit and certainly better than doing nothing, it won't boost your metabolic rate or burn a ton of calories unless you change it up frequently and challenge yourself. By that, I mean increasing/decreasing speed, elevation, and duration. This is true for all of your workouts. It's important to get the heart rate up, and keep it up, but build short recovery segments into your workouts to allow the heart to stay in your target range. **NOTE: It is recommended that you exercise within 55 to 85 percent of your maximum heart rate for at least 20 to 30 minutes to get the best results from aerobic exercise. The MHR (maximum heart rate is roughly calculated as 220 minus your age), and is the upper limit of what your cardiovascular system can handle during physical activity.**

This is also why circuit training is so effective. Combining strength training with short bursts of aerobic activity will do wonders for boosting your metabolism and varying your routine so you won't get bored.

In the case of your treadmill walking for example, start with a five minute warm-up at 2.0-2.5 mph. Then do two minute intervals at 3.0-3.5 (depending on your tolerance, you may be able to work up to 4.0-4.5 mph. Anything faster than that will likely push you into jogging mode). Increase your speed or change your elevation each time, and try to stick it out for at least thirty minutes. Allow yourself a five minute cool down, and stretch afterward to prevent injury. Walking backwards on the treadmill (holding onto the handrails) at 1.0 mph for the last few minutes is an excellent way to "unwind" the muscles, cool down, and avoid soreness. The key is to switch it up and keep your body guessing and adapting.

NOTE: Learn how to take your pulse and know your MHR (maximum heart rate). Never "work through" chest pain, and stop if you become short of breath or can't hold a conversation during the workout. Muscle soreness, fatigue, and feeling the "burn" won't kill you, but a heart attack will. Use common sense and consult your physician before beginning any new exercise program.

- **Make ADLs (activities of daily living) work for you.** If formal exercise isn't your bag, simply increasing your daily activity level can easily add up to your 250 extra calories/day burn. Consider the following activities (calories measured in per hour units):

Moving boxes (packing and unpacking) = 191 calories
Vacuuming = 119 calories
Cleaning the house = 102 calories
Playing with the kids (moderate activity level) = 136 calories

Mowing the lawn = 205 calories
Raking leaves = 147 calories
Gardening or weeding = 153 calories
Strolling = 103 calories
Biking to work (on a flat surface) = 220 calories

Before we leave Mary Jane to set up her goals and revamp her eating habits, there's one more topic I'd like to address here.

Body Image

From the time we are born, we are learning about ourselves through the people and world around us. Doling out nicknames like "chunky monkey" to our infant child or describing a toddler as "chubby" are the beginning of a lifelong battle with body image and poor self-esteem. Words are powerful! Even well-meaning adults can cause deep wounds through careless use of language and teasing that can leave scars for a lifetime. If we are given negative messages about ourselves for long enough, they become the truth that defines us.

These negative messages, along with the barrage of images we are bombarded by from the media, movies, and magazines create deeply rooted beliefs about what is "normal" and how we stack up against others. In an environment where perfection is a requirement for being loved and admired, one can see why most of us come away with the impression that we are neither loved nor admired, since we are clearly imperfect. Once these beliefs are ingrained in our psyche, they cloud our perceptions of what is real and true. It's easy to understand how unrealistic expectations of ourselves and others becomes the lens through which we see the world. From eating disorders to obesity, what our brains have been repeatedly fed has created a dysfunctional self-image for millions of people.

Reading beauty magazines will only make you feel ugly.

STOP the madness! Accept that we are all individuals and that each of us is perfectly imperfect in our own way. Learning to love yourself as you are is the first step to loving yourself enough to make positive changes in your life. That may sound contradictory, but in fact, until we can accept and love ourselves today, we will continue to feel undeserving and have no clue as to how to make healthy choices for our future. We will remain forever stuck in that mindset of "I'm fat, I'm stupid," or "I'm undeserving of…" you fill in the blank.

Washing our minds clean of these messages takes time, effort, and a real commitment. I had a counselor once who assigned me some homework that I thought was ridiculous and unnecessary. After all, I didn't have low self-esteem. I merely made horrible choices in relationships because I'd had a troubled childhood and poor role models for healthy relationships. My outgoing, sunshiny personality clearly meant that I had a healthy self-image. Right? Um…no. My teen years of being anorexic and bulimic and my alcohol and drug use probably should have clued me in. Oh, Denial be thy name.

The assignment required me to find a picture of myself as a small child, hang it on my mirror, and every day, I was told to look at that picture and say, **"I love you and I'm going to take care of you today."**

At first, I thought this a simple but useless exercise. Until I realized how hard it was to do. At first, I couldn't say the words at all. I'd just stare at the picture and feel an incredible sadness and sense of loss. Then the sadness turned to frustration and anger. Why couldn't I say the words? After days of tormenting myself with that unanswerable question, I forced myself to say it. Through gritted teeth, I recited the words, but I couldn't allow myself to truly connect to their meaning. Did I truly NOT love myself? Was I unwilling to take care of myself and do what was in my best interest?

It was months later, after reciting the meaningless words daily, that finally one day, I realized it was true. I did love that little girl. I did want to take care of her. And I wanted more than anything to make her feel safe. Tears flooded my eyes and my heart broke into a million pieces. I realized I'd left that child locked away inside me in order to protect her, but in doing so, I'd denied her existence. I had denied she had needs, wants, hopes, and dreams. Needless to say, that was a pivotal moment in life for me. Mending my heart and retraining my thinking took time, heart wrenching honesty, and a very good counselor. But the healing that took place after that one realization was nothing short of miraculous. I recommend the exercise to anyone struggling with self-worth and body image issues.

After you've mastered the "I love you and I'm going to take care of you today," try posting these messages wherever you'll see them on a daily basis, say them out loud, and say them until you mean them.

Be who you are; love who you are.
Love and nurture yourself with every choice you make.
Guilt is an overdeveloped sense of responsibility and a useless emotion. Get rid of it!
Beauty is found, not on the surface of a painting, but in its layers. (The same is true for us.)
Being different is what makes me uniquely qualified to pave the way for change.
The more I learn to love myself, the more love I have to share with the world.
My physical being does not define me.
I am worthy of being loved.

The only way to override the old messages that no longer serve you is to bombard yourself with new ones. Make up your own positive messages, say them out loud and often, and watch the transformation unfold.

CHAPTER 7

IMPORTANCE OF SLEEP

Sleep deprivation is a public health epidemic!

Adequate SLEEP is a MUST.

Habitually depriving ourselves of sleep (intentionally or unintentionally), contributes to a plethora of physical, psychological, emotional, and even social problems. Poor sleep habits increase risk factors for heart disease, high blood pressure, and Type-2 Diabetes as well as compromise cell repair and overall vitality (dark circles and wrinkles anyone?). Lack of sleep can weaken the immune system, contribute to depression, increase irritability and anxiety, and shorten life expectancy. Thousands of lives per year are lost to car accidents and injuries caused by sleep deprivation. I, myself, almost lost my life to falling asleep at the wheel and hitting a tree at 40 mph. I had just come back from an overseas trip and didn't account for the power of jet lag. Thank God I didn't kill anyone else or suffer any crippling injuries. Talk about a wake-up call!

More to the point for our original discussion on conquering your metabolism, inadequate sleep is a huge contributor to obesity, hormonal imbalances, and chronic inflammatory conditions (a factor in numerous diseases, including cancer). Sleeplessness kills, but before it kills you, it will make you fat.

Without adequate rest and recovery, our quality of life and ability to function optimally are greatly diminished.

If you suffer from insomnia, sleep apnea, or some other sleep disorder that's interfering with your ability to get a good night's sleep (that includes getting a good mattress and earplugs as needed), do something about it. See your doctor for a sleep study or appropriate medications for your condition. Be willing to change your habits. If you really want to take some responsibility, admit all the things you're doing to sabotage your sleep.

Are you burning the candle at both ends to meet those deadlines? Worrying and obsessing about things over which you have no control? Revving up your adrenal gland by watching action-packed television until the wee hours? These are all self-defeating activities that will put you on the road to ruin.

Here are my best tips for mastering the sleep monster:

- Get adequate exercise/movement throughout the day to curb restless sleep at night.
- For just one week, settle on an absolute bedtime and stick to it, even if you don't feel tired.
- Try shutting down the computer and TV at least an hour before bed. Read instead.
- Lower the lights in your home in the evenings, especially around the computer so your mind starts to wind down and signal the end of your workday.

- Soak in a hot bath with Epsom salts and lavender essential oil before you settle in for the night, or put a few drops of lavender on a tissue and tuck it into your pillowcase. (If you get stuffy at night or are suffering from a cold, try a few drops of eucalyptus on a tissue tucked into the pillowcase instead.)
- Take some deep breaths and progressively relax your limbs, working from feet to head.
- Try a cup of chamomile tea an hour or so before you go to sleep. If you're worried it will keep you up in trips to the bathroom, skip the tea and opt for a slice of turkey before bed. **(No nitrites, please. Applegate makes high quality uncured cold meats without nitrites).** The tryptophan can trigger sleep hormones, while the protein will break down slowly through the night and aid in cell repair. Warm milk has the same effect.

I manage my sleep with a combination of yoga, deep breathing, and herbal remedies (chamomile tea knocks me out but doesn't make me feel groggy in the morning). I also take a daily multi-vitamin specifically for menopausal women who often have difficulty with sleep due to fluctuating hormones. Herbal remedies or calcium/magnesium supplements can help, as well as products such as melatonin or other over the counter sleep aids. Ask your doctor or naturopath for recommendations.

Princess and the Pea Syndrome:
If you're a bit sensitive like me or are living with chronic pain, you may find it difficult to find a comfortable position in which to sleep. You toss and turn like a writhing bag of snakes and punch the pillow to get it just right, only to have to change positions five more times before finally drifting off. I call this the Princess and the Pea Syndrome. Nothing seems to work to make sleeping comfortable, and the more agitated you are about NOT sleeping, the worse the situation becomes.

I'm not talking about Restless Leg Syndrome (RLS), which effects 10% of Americans and is a neurological disorder characterized by unpleasant sensations in the legs and an uncomfortable urge to move them when at rest in an effort to relieve these feelings. Sensations of burning, creeping, tugging, or as if insects are crawling inside the legs are indicators of RLS. These paresthesia's (abnormal sensations) can range in severity from uncomfortable to irritating to downright painful, and may require medication to manage. I'll note here that there are several herbal remedies that can also treat this condition quite effectively, so please consult your physician or naturopath to discuss your options if you think you have RLS.

What about those leg cramps? Ouch! A well placed foot, calf, or hamstring cramp in the middle of the night can drive you out of sleep and have you howling in pain as if you've been shot. The only way to alleviate them once they're in full blown cramp mode is to get up and stretch the muscle. Massaging the arch of the foot, forcing the heel down to the floor, or bending forward with your leg straight to stretch out a hamstring cramp will give you temporary relief but wouldn't it be nice not to get them at all?

There are several known contributors to leg cramps, but narrowing down the culprit takes some experimentation. Lack of proper hydration is a good place to start. See if reducing your caffeine intake and increasing your water consumption makes a difference before moving on to adding supplements like calcium/magnesium or potassium. Sometimes it's as simple as eating a few bites of a banana before bed (potassium has been shown to help reduce leg cramps), or keeping a homemade brew of apple cider vinegar, ginger, and garlic juice next to the bed and taking a teaspoon before settling in for the night. This old Amish recipe works! It's even available online. Another old folk remedy is placing a bar of soap at the bottom of the bed under the sheets. I've never tried it, but I've heard it works. Of course, daily stretching and an occasional massage can be of tremendous benefit as well. Whatever it takes to get those leg cramps under control, figure it out. You need a good night's sleep.

More tips for getting comfy:

Do you wake up out of alignment, creaky, and walking like you're ninety years old for the first five minutes of your day? Positioning for successful sleep is challenging, but here are my best solutions for helping you maintain proper alignment so you don't feel like humpty dumpty every morning.

- **Invest in a good mattress.** In keeping with our fairy tale theme, Goldilocks had to try a few beds before settling on the one that was "just right." But mattresses are expensive and lying on one for ten minutes in the store doesn't give you a clear indication of how your body will react after eight hours—or eight months of sleeping on said mattress. The thing is, our bodies change over time, and even day to day, we might need more or less support. For this reason alone, adjustable mattresses make the most sense to me. I slept on a horrible mattress for years (one that was perfect for my husband), until I just couldn't do it anymore. I proceeded to buy a mattress that felt good to me, and he was nearly crippled after a few months of sleeping on it. We finally invested in an adjustable air mattress with dual controls and are both much happier for it. Do some research. The big name brands aren't the only game in town, and we were able to find a great setup for about half the price of the leading competitor.
- **Use pillow supports** between the knees and under your top arm if you are a side sleeper. They make full-length body pillows that are perfect for this but you might want to experiment first with the pillows you have. The pillow between the knees takes pressure off the low back and hips and keeps the spine in proper alignment. Tucking a pillow under the arm supports the upper back, shoulders, and neck and can alleviate the middle of the night numbness and tingling in the hands, which is often caused by nerve compression at the neck, shoulder, or wrist. (Wearing wrist braces at night can also be helpful if carpal tunnel is the culprit.)
Addendum: To relieve numbness and tingling in the hand, try stretching the shoulder and chest by straightening the arm, reaching behind you with palm up and thumb pointing back. Hold and breathe deeply for about 20-30 seconds.
- **If you sleep on your back**, tuck a pillow under your knees, and if you are a **stomach sleeper** (the worst position for your neck and back, by the way), be sure to tuck a pillow under your hips/belly to avoid hyperextension of the spine.
- **Temperature control and blanket hogging.** If you share your bed with man or beast, you probably already know where this is going. My husband is a furnace. I, on the other hand, suffer from cold feet from September to June living here in the Northeast. You'd think we'd be a perfect match, right? We were—and still are in many ways—but then those damn night sweats and hot flashes struck. Ugh! First I'm cold, then I'm hot. We like it cool in the house at night (average winter temp is about 55 degrees in our old farm house).

The blankets were on…then off…one leg out…socks on…socks off…you get the picture. Until I purchased a bed warmer. Best investment EVER! I bought a table warmer at the massage school, which fits a massage table so it only covers my side of the bed. I turn it on for a half hour before I go to bed so when I get in at night, the bed is nice and toasty. It's on a timer so it goes off by the time I've fallen asleep. My husband and I also each have our own blanket so I don't disturb him with my middle of the night "blanket dance."

It takes experimentation, patience, and a "MacGyver" attitude to find what works, but we spend nearly a third of our lives in bed sleeping. Isn't it worth it to make it the best experience it can be?

Last NOTE on sleep: While it's true that children and young adults require more sleep (10-12 hours per night), and that the average adult under the age of sixty-five should shoot for about 7-9, older folks tend to require slightly less, and do fine on 6-7 hours. I suspect that those of you who are averaging under six hours per night—you know who you are—need to take a closer look at the cost to your health. Your life truly does depend upon it!

CHAPTER 8

ERGONOMICS 101

You're eating right, getting more sleep, and jumping into a new lifestyle. You'd be loving it if it weren't for that eight to ten hours you are "required" to put in at your desk every day. Those, who by circumstance or choice, are spending a third of your life sitting behind a desk and computer, this section is for you. It may not be within your control to work less hours, take more breaks, or ignore deadlines. But if you're going to spend a third of your life at your desk, it better be comfortable and ergonomically sound.

Correct desk and chair height/placement

There's a science to workstation set up called Ergonomics, which is based on biomechanics. Studying the way in which work related activities stress the body, we've come to understand how to correct and alleviate potential problems. Proper alignment of the spine is essential for maintaining muscle balance—and vice versa. Knowing how to apply the necessary forces and make changes to adapt requires specialized research. It's important to note, however, that ergonomics is a fairly new concept and new information comes out frequently regarding what's right for us and what hasn't worked out so well.

Guidelines should be adapted to the particular needs of the person and are not set in stone. What works for you may not work for someone else.

The recommended baseline parameters are as follows:
- Your screen should be a minimum of 20 inches from you. This may vary slightly depending on visual acuity.
- Place the center of the screen at approximately a 15 degree angle down from your eyes with your neck only slightly bent but keeping your ears in line with your shoulders.
- Position your keyboard slightly below the elbow (90-100 degree angle) and your mouse at the same height as, and close by, your keyboard. Have your keyboard in a flat position (elevating the back higher than the front will cause wrist problems). Use wrist rests only for resting and NOT while typing or mousing.
- Take frequent breaks. Ten minutes for every hour of work and 30 second micro-breaks every 10 minutes is a good schedule. Stretch during your breaks.

The following guidelines are an accepted industry standard.

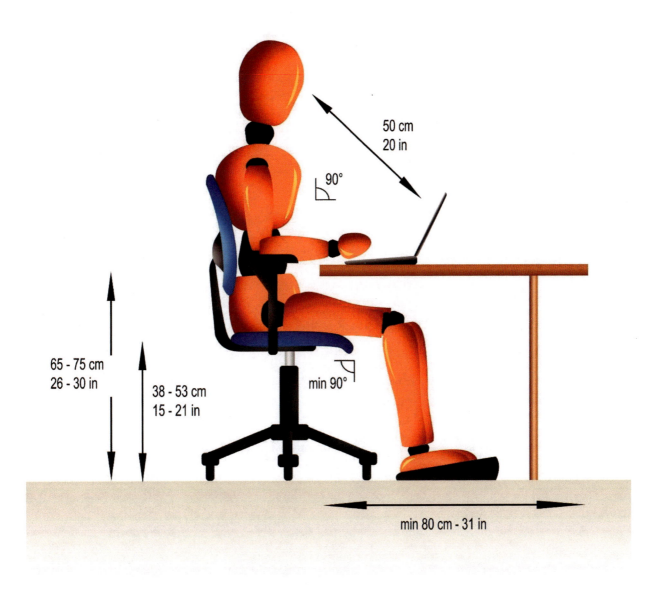

Fig. 6 Correct Desk Ergonomics

Having said that, it's important to take into consideration the size and body type of a person and individual preferences for comfort. Set at the correct height, arm rests offer support for the neck and upper back by taking the weight of the upper extremities. Wrist rests (not shown in this graphic) are essential for both your keyboard and mouse pad. I think it's also important to note that new research by ophthalmologists suggests that keeping the eyes slightly downward and looking at a tilted screen are better and more natural on the eyes than staring straight ahead. Try lowering your screen slightly and tilting it away from you as suggested above.
This graphic has the person working from a laptop sized computer rather than a larger desk top screen, which requires the head to be too far forward for my liking.

Find what works for you, but be sure to consider posture, alignment, and your individual comfort.

Finding the right chair

Try as many chairs as you can find at different stores. IKEA, Staples, and Office Max have a variety of choices, and even your local BJ's or Costco can have some great office chairs at reasonable prices. Sit in them, adjust them to your height according to the graphic above, and choose the one that makes you feel like you're sitting on a cloud. You'll know it when you find it. A comfortable, supportive chair is essential for your longevity in the sitting business.

A few extra tips: The more adjustable your chair is, the better, since your body will change over time.
- When you sit in your prospective new chair, adjust the seat height to make sure your feet are flat on the floor. (Consider a foot rest if your desk height and the rest of your setup doesn't allow you to put your feet flat. Plan to move your feet often and avoid crossing your ankles.)
- Use a high backed chair so your lower back and shoulder blades are supported if possible.
- Allow 1-3 inches between the edge of the seat and the back of your knees.
- Have your hips slightly higher than your knees (100-110 degree angle at the hips is acceptable). The picture above has the hips and elbows at 90 degree angles. **The angle should be slightly more than that to be optimal.**
- Arm rests are set so your arms hang naturally and shoulders relax down and back.
- Make sure you have adequate leg room under your desk.

MacGyver Style: If a new chair isn't in your budget right now, and you have a chair that suits your needs but is lacking in the support department, consider using a back support. Back pillows come in all shapes, sizes, and prices. You may have to try a few before you find the right one. Supports made of a flexible webbing are nice for car and office as they breathe well and offer firm but comfortable support. I've seen them in places like Bed Bath and Beyond, Target, and Walmart. In a pinch, fold a bath towel in half, then in half again and roll it to make a nice comfortable and no cost lumbar support which you will place just below the waistline.

Less MacGyver and more James Bond: If you want to invest a couple hundred dollars in a portable seat you can take to conferences or workshops and apply to any chair to make it your own, check out the Relax Your Back Store or local Brookstone Store for something more substantial.

Accessories
Computer, mouse, and keyboard considerations

Dual, and even triple monitor set-ups are all the rage. My husband, who is an engineer and all around tech-spert, has done a wonderful job outfitting me with the latest and greatest in computers and gadgetry. I currently have two monitors, which allows me to have several documents open simultaneously, check on my email as needed, or work between multiple documents should the need arise. This works outstandingly for me as a writer and multi-tasker. It completely eliminates the need for a document stand or secondary device. My main screen is directly in front of me and the second screen is slightly off to my left. The one caveat I would include here is that you need to make sure you move your "active" document to the screen in front of you to avoid prolonged poor positioning of the head. I sometimes forget to do this until my neck starts squealing from being turned to the left for too long. In my next office set-up, I'll have three screens as well as an alternative standing desk. We'll see how I adapt.

As was pointed out in the general considerations of ergonomic desk set up, your mouse should be at the same height as your keyboard and within a close and comfortable reach. Nothing will crank up your neck, shoulder, and wrist pain faster than reaching too far for your mouse. Consider a roller mouse to reduce stress on the hand and wrist. Remember to take your hand off the mouse when you're reading or not using it immediately. We often forget to release our hand from the mouse when we're in the groove and not paying attention. **Keep your wrists straight.** Any angle beyond neutral is going to eventually cause you problems.

Don't Forget Lighting

Proper lighting makes a huge difference in productivity, mood, and energy. When setting up your home office, you'll want your space to be pleasant, free from distraction, and functional. Natural lighting is always best, so if you can set up your desk near a window to capitalize on this, all the better—as long as it isn't creating glare on your computer screen. Having a view to the outdoors also has a tremendous effect on attitude and frame of mind. You'll feel less cooped up if you have access to a pleasant view or enjoy some sunlight.

If your desk isn't near a window, take time during the day to walk around outside, even if it means adding a walk at lunchtime or spending your break time in the nearest "green area." Connecting with nature is one of the most effective solutions for rejuvenating yourself after hours at the computer.

When considering home office lighting, start with overhead lights. There are some great options for track and recessed lighting that are non-fluorescent and soft on the eyes. LED technology has come a long way. Most LEDs are now energy efficient, dimmable, and much less disruptive to vision.

Fluorescent lights? I feel for you. There's not much you can do to combat them directly, but see if it's possible to have them turned off during the day, or add a shield to the fixture covering the bulbs. Fluorescent lights are a migraine trigger! Avoid them whenever possible.

Ambient light, also called, corrective lighting, is just as important as having your workspace well lit. Ambient light fills in the surrounding area with a soothing glow for an aesthetic and comfortable atmosphere, adding to the supportive feel of the environment. Rope lights, shaded lamps that diffuse light in the back ground, or small under desk lights can be just the right fillers that help reduce glare and need for bright overhead lighting. Don't forget to consider placement, and whether a low desk height or high light will work best with your setup.

Wrist rests, foot rests, and Thera-canes, oh my!

Many keyboards and mouse pads come with built in wrist rests to help you maintain neutral alignment and support the wrist. This becomes important for avoiding carpal tunnel syndrome, which can occur with excessive and repetitive motions of the wrist and fingers or prolonged pressure over the carpal tunnel which houses the nerves innervating the hand and wrist.

Tendons which control movement of the fingers and wrist are held in place by a band of fibrous connective tissue called a retinaculum, which wraps around the wrist. If tendons become inflamed due to overuse, are compressed by the retinaculum, or are at a biomechanical disadvantage because of improper alignment—pain, weakness, or nerve impingement (characterized by numbness and tingling) may occur. That's not to say the symptoms might not be coming from higher up, such as is the case with cervical disc herniation or thoracic outlet syndrome, but the first plan of attack to avoiding these debilitating conditions is to check that you have proper support under your wrists. Don't keep your wrists on the rests while typing or using your mouse. Continuous pressure over the carpal tunnel is what leads to compression and inflammation.

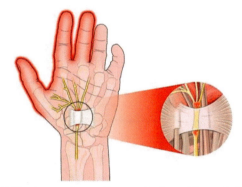

Fig. 7 Retinaculum Constricting Carpal Tunnel

If you've done all you can to insure that your desk and chair height are optimal for offering good spinal alignment and upper extremity positioning, your monitor, mouse, and keyboard are adjusted correctly, but your feet don't quite sit flat on the floor, consider a foot rest as well. These are easy to find in office supply stores, or you can certainly order one online at a reasonable price, but if you need to scrimp on office supplies, this is one you could easily MacGyver. Any wedge-shaped block of wood will do the trick. Even a fairly flat, hard pillow or cushion will work.

I use one of my old wedge shaped lap desks which was an abysmal failure since it turned out to be not quite the right height for me and not adjustable. It works perfectly, however, as a foot rest.

You'll probably have to play around with a lot of options and likely even have many blunders until you get your office space set exactly right for you, but don't give up trying to tweak it to perfection. If you're experiencing pain while at your desk, re-examine your workstation. Even the smallest changes can have a tremendous impact.

One more essential tool in my self-care office arsenal is a **Thera-cane** (also known as a "back buddy"). It's a large S-shaped hook made from composite plastic. There are several small, round, knob-like appendages (some are slightly pointed), that stick out. You'll use the Thera-cane to root out and treat your own trigger points, which ultimately, are the likely culprits for much of your neck and back pain.

A trigger point is a group of irritated nerve endings in a muscle. Due to overuse, prolonged tension, or other stresses, muscles stay tight, compressing on the blood vessels whose job it is to bring fresh blood supply to the muscle fibers and carry away waste products. When those waste products build up, toxins remain in the tissue, causing inflammation and irritation. Over time, those trigger points become chronic and cause referred pain to other areas of the body.

The headache you're experiencing after sitting too long at the computer may be emanating from a trigger point in your rhomboids or mid traps (shoulder blade area). You can rest the Thera-cane over your shoulder and press into the trigger points to aid in releasing them. Be gentle. It doesn't take much pressure once you've found the right spots. Consistent treatment of trigger points can alleviate much of your pain and improve the circulation to your postural muscles as well as reduce chronic headaches, fatigue, and range of motion restriction. I'll be addressing this further in the chapter on **TREATMENT**.

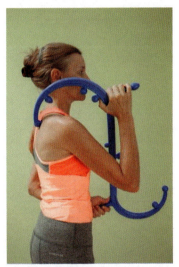

Fig. 8 Thera Cane on Levator Scapulae T.P.

You can pick up one of these handy-dandy Thera-canes online for about $30. It's well-worth the investment. The Thera-cane is easy to use, convenient, and extremely effective at working out knots of tension wherever they might arise. At least a few times a week, I sit with my Thera-cane (usually while I'm watching TV), and I work on the trigger points in my neck, shoulders, upper back, and hips. It takes a little practice to find them and to know exactly how much pressure to exert to gain the desired effect, but I can't recommend this self-care tool highly enough. It's a life saver!

NOTE: You'll know you're on a trigger point when you hit a spot that is significantly tender and radiates pain outward from the general area. Sensation may travel upward, downward, or outward, or you may feel it remotely. (I often feel pain behind my ear when I hit a trigger point on my upper trapezius or feel as if I have an icepick in my eye when I focus a bit of pressure on my sub occipital muscles at the base of my skull.)

Trigger points can be painful, but releasing them is key to reducing your pain and improving your function, so breathe through them and use your judgment about working within your tolerance. We aren't leaving marks here, people, so ere on the side of caution.

Another thing that helps tremendously is adding movement to your trigger point release. For instance, once you find a trigger point in your neck or upper back, slowly turn your head side to side, shrug and roll your shoulder slowly, or otherwise try to get a little deeper into the release. It only requires a small amount of movement, but the payoff is big. There are some excellent resources regarding trigger point therapy online. I'll talk more about this in the section on **TREATMENT**.

Air Quality Matters

Air quality and ventilation are also important and often overlooked considerations. Nothing saps your energy or depresses a person more than being stuck in a stuffy, dirty, dingy office space with poor ventilation and dusty carpets. Changing air conditioning and heating duct filters on a routine basis will keep dust down and aid in reducing allergens, but nothing improves the atmosphere more than a good cleaning. You spend an inordinate amount of time at your office space, so allowing dust bunnies to collect isn't in the best interest of your lungs—or your mood. Declutter and dust your space often.

Develop the habit at the end of your day of clearing your desk of unnecessary paperwork, books, and food items that might attract critters. (You don't want mice, ants, or other invaders leaving you presents that can make you sick.) A clean work environment boosts your energy, mood, and productivity. You'll breathe better, and being more organized will leave you less stressed. Reduce exposure to chemicals by using all natural cleaning products and try sprinkling a bit of baking soda on carpets as you vacuum to eliminate odors. Keep plants watered and healthy and they will assist you in keeping the air clean.

A NOTE ON FENG SHUI: Feng Shui is the art of harmonizing people with their environment. Chinese philosophy suggests that we are connected to—and thereby affected by—everything around us. How we arrange our furnishings, what artwork we choose, and the color scheme of our surroundings all have a direct effect on our mood, energy level, and productivity. I'm sure you've walked into homes or offices that were drab, cluttered, and depressing. You might not have even noticed why, but you sensed the negativity or lack of positive energy flow. Then again, you've probably walked into a room and felt an immediate positive shift in your energy when confronted with a warm and welcoming atmosphere, where furnishings were placed just so, the lighting wasn't overpowering, and the colors were soothing. Feng Shui matters.

Strategically placing plants, crystals, or other energy promoting items around our home and office can make a significant difference in how we feel. Even the location of these items (the Northwest corner of a room, for instance, is the money and prosperity center) can improve the quality of our energy. There are many online resources for easy to implement changes you can incorporate into your décor to optimize the flow of positive energy around you. It's well worth educating yourself on the subject

and exploring the possibilities.

Optimizing your workspace can take time, money, and lots of trial and error before you find what works best for you, but believe me, it's worth every penny and every minute it takes to create a healthy environment for yourself. If you're spending a third of your life there, you'll want it to fit your needs and effect you positively. To bring us back around to our fairy tale motif, whether it's finding the right chair, lumbar support, or foot rest, sometimes, you have to kiss a lot of frogs before you find your prince.

CHAPTER 9

EXERCISE BASICS

Basics of Breathing

Speaking of air quality, when was the last time you took a deep breath? Oxygen is the most vital nutrient our bodies require. We can survive without food or water for days, but without oxygen, we will die within a few minutes. Ever notice that you tend to hold your breath when you're stressed? For most of our day, without giving it much thought, we breathe shallowly into our chest and never quite take a deep enough breath to fill our lungs. This shallow chest breathing is part of our fight or flight response, and though helpful when we are trying to escape a predator, does us no favors in our day to day desk dwelling lifestyle. Over time, shallow breathing can lead to reduced oxygen uptake, fatigue, headache, increased muscle tension, and heart problems, etc. Most of the time, we aren't aware of our breathing, so we don't even realize we're doing this…another excellent reason to practice *mindfulness*.

There are many ways to improve the quality of our breathing and change old patterns that have been adopted through years of chronic stress, poor posture, and lack of awareness. The practice of Pranayama, yogic breathing, is one way. Find a class, buy a DVD, or just look it up on YouTube. There is plenty of information on different techniques, but it's in your best interest to learn HOW to breathe properly. Practice it until it becomes second nature. Tai Chi and Qi Gong are other excellent resources for learning breath work and will change your life! Imagine being able to find a calm center inside yourself with just a single breath while in the midst of a chaotic family gathering, a frustrating traffic jam, or a stressful board meeting.

Try this exercise:
1) Sit up straight, elongate your spine, and lift the crown of your head skyward.
2) Simply sit and notice your breathing for about thirty seconds.
3) Now, draw in a slow, deep breath through your nose, noticing the path it takes in your body.
4) Allow the breath to expand your chest, fill your lungs, and sink into your belly. Don't worry if it doesn't quite reach all the way down on the first or second try. (It may take many breaths before you can relax enough to breathe deeply).
5) Release the breath slowly through your mouth as if blowing it out through a straw.

Repeat this cleansing breath three times.

Now we'll try breathing in and out through the nose. In yoga this is called Ujjayi breath (sometimes called "victorious breathing" or "ocean breath") and is similar to diaphragmatic breathing.

1) This might feel backward and slightly counter-intuitive at first, but practice makes perfect. Allow the breath to seep in through the nose, fill the belly, rise to the lower rib cage, and then up into the upper chest and throat. Release the breath slowly in reverse.

2) Now try it while gently constricting your throat (the glottis, or muscle in your throat that narrows the opening can be gently contracted) as you inhale and exhale. It's as if you are sighing with your mouth closed and will make a "rushing" sound. (Have you ever observed your dog or cat breathing in this manner when they sleep? Animals breathe diaphragmatically on a routine basis because it relaxes their nervous system and oxygenates their bodies, just as it will do for us. They do this instinctively and don't allow stress to disturb their Zen. There is much to be learned from the animal kingdom.)
3) Continue with five to ten breaths, keeping in mind that you want to draw the breath in and release it slowly at the same rate. You may want to try inhaling for a count of five and exhaling for a count of five, gradually increasing the time as you're able to draw deeper breaths. These slow steady breaths will center and re-energize your mind.

NOTE: If you can't quite master the concept of Ujjayi breathing, there are plenty of YouTube videos that walk you through the technique and demonstrate it for you. Even better is to take a pranayama class and learn to cultivate the power of breath work.

Just think of how much more productive you would be if you took even a five minute break every few hours and did this exercise. I challenge you to set a timer and do this at least three times a day every day for a week. You will see immediate benefits in that you will feel calmer and more in control of your thoughts and emotions. You will also feel more relaxed and alert. Train yourself to do this throughout your day.

Finding Time is Making Time

Any amount of increased activity will go a long way toward overcoming your sedentary lifestyle and fighting the battle of the bulge, but to see real results, consistency and intensity are key.

You don't have to love exercise. You just have to hate being out of shape more than you hate getting into shape.

By "vigorous" exercise, as I mentioned earlier, I mean sweating, getting your heart rate up, and making your muscles work for 30 minutes a day five days per week. Mix it up. It can be a combination of aerobic activity, light strength training, or plyometric exercise. Also don't discount the benefits of activity based workouts like kayaking, biking, hiking, tennis, or taking a dance class—whatever gets you out of your head and into your body for at least a half hour every day.

Exercise is essential to a balanced, healthy life. There is no way around it.

Please consult a physician before beginning an exercise routine and:
START SLOW.

If you need gentler, lower impact activities; swimming, Tai Chi, Qi Gong, gentle yoga, or Pilates might help to get you fit enough for more strenuous pursuits. Just don't give in to the idea of **all** or **nothing**. Do something…anything…but learn to do it correctly and commit to doing it consistently.

Daily exercise is something you must do for the rest of your life, so find activities you enjoy and become proficient with them. There is no race to the finish line here, but you must make a commitment to yourself to make exercise a priority. Developing a routine takes time, but it's clearly one of the most impactful choices you can make for optimal physical and mental well-being and is a cornerstone to weight management.

For example, I work my day job as a massage therapist and personal trainer three to four days per week. It sounds like I'd get a lot of exercise, but in reality, giving massages is not terribly demanding for me. My body is conditioned and used to performing this activity so I don't include it as exercise. The same with training. I might demonstrate an activity now and then, but mostly I'm instructing, and definitely not working up a sweat. That means that on the days I work from home (my sedentary writing life takes up an additional thirty to forty hours a week or more), I follow a routine.

On those days at home I get up around 7:00 a.m. (I'm a night owl so I don't get to bed until 11:30 or midnight, but I still try for at least seven hours of sleep), don my workout duds, fill my water bottle, and break my nighttime fast. I'll have a piece of fruit or a few bites of protein (a couple spoons full of low fat cottage cheese or yogurt works well to tide me over until breakfast.) Then I sit down to go through my emails, take care of any promotional responsibilities, and check in with my social media sites. This can take anywhere from 1-2 hours, depending on how much I need to attend to. I set my internal timer to remind me to do some shoulder shrugs and wrist and neck stretches at the half hour marks. **If you need to set a timer, do it.**

On the other hand, if you're an early morning writer, and most creative first thing, this two hours (even with breaks every half hour) can get you that 1000 words a day word count quota most writers strive for. I'm not one of those who can jump out of bed and hit the treadmill or force my creative brain to kick into high gear. I'm also not a coffee drinker, but if you are, now's the time to enjoy your wakeup call. By 9:00, whether I'm done or not, I get up and prepare to exercise.

I'm already dressed, my blood sugar is level, and I've got my first water bottle several ounces down by now. I remind myself adamantly that I can do anything for 30 minutes. I slap in a DVD, line up my weights, rollout my mat, and before I know it, it's over and I feel like I just climbed a mountain. Sweaty but invigorated, I feel as if I can tackle anything that comes my way for the rest of the day. If I want to mix it up, or need a quick 20 minute routine, I throw in a kickboxing video or do my own heavy bag routine.

As I said before, there are a ton of options when it comes to video workouts. It can be overwhelming to find what's right for you, but be patient, do your homework, and then pick your poison.

My advice to those who are not "athletic" or who fear injury:

Consult a personal trainer if you've never lifted weights, or try any one of a thousand "beginner" DVDs on the market to get you going on a path to learning about your body and how it responds to movement of all kinds. Become proficient at various types of exercise so you have plenty of choices. Be willing to try something new. Pilates, yoga, and even Zumba are fun ways to explore just what that body of yours is capable of. Join a class, start slow, but commit to getting on board with exercise. Remember…NO EXCUSES! **Everyone can do *something*.**

Incidentally, you won't die from exercise induced sweating. And as long as you **listen to your body, focus on your breath, and employ your common sense**, you'll be fine. You'll also be less likely to injure yourself and more likely to engage in exercise on a regular basis if you find the right exercise routine for you. **The idea is to find a way to not equate exercise with drudgery.**

By the same token, if you aren't willing to work up a sweat, your results will be less pronounced and goals will take longer to achieve. Remember that weight management and health maintenance are a lifelong pursuit. You don't have to do it all today, but every step you take toward improving the quality of your life through daily exercise and healthy eating will have a positive impact.

If you want to go the exercise video route—the least expensive and most convenient way to get started—here are some suggestions:

- Choose the appropriate fitness level for you and pick something you'll enjoy doing over and over again. Gaiam offers many choices for beginner workouts in Yoga and Pilates from great instructors like Rodney Yee and Sean Corn, experts in the field with years of experience.
- Make sure your DVD of choice has an instructional segment and offers several shorter workouts so you have multiple options on any given day, depending on time limitations or how you're feeling that day. You don't want to give yourself any excuse to skip out on your workout.
- Go on **exercisevideosreviews.com** to see what's available and how one stacks up against others.
- Create an exercise space for yourself. It doesn't take much room, but you'll want easy access to your weights, mat, and TV. Again, you want to make it easy to say YES to exercise.
- Wear the proper clothing. You don't have to have the latest in yoga fashion, but wear comfortable, stretchable, breathable clothing, good shoes, and ladies—a sports bra. Have water available and set yourself up for success by previewing your video to see if there are exercises you can't do or if there is someone on stage offering a modified version. Don't worry about keeping up. Do what you can.
- The FIRM's Super Body Sculpt series and all the "For Dummies" videos are excellent for teaching good form and setting you on the right track.
- For more advanced exercisers who are generally in good health and looking for someone to kick their butts back into shape, try Jillian Michael's 90 Day Body Revolution DVDs, P90X, or the Beach Body DVD series. These are all excellent for getting great results, but you have to be willing to work hard and stick with it to see the results you want.
- Mix it up. Your body will adapt to a new routine quickly, so I recommend cross-training by varying your workout routines frequently. At the very least, switch up your routine every 6-8 weeks to keep your body guessing and adapting.

If you find that you can't get a workout in at home because:

a) There are too many demands on your attention (kids, dogs, and spouses need to eat)
b) You have difficulty focusing on exercise when you feel you should be doing other things at home (like dishes, laundry, or lawn care).
c) You simply hate workout videos and prefer a gym setting.

By all means, join a gym.

It doesn't have to be the fancy place with all the amenities that costs an arm and leg. There are plenty of small gyms and inexpensive alternatives as low as $10 per month. Some even have daycare available so you can bring the kids along. Once you commit, you need to put it on your schedule as a non-negotiable appointment. Whatever else you do that day is not as important as your health. Keep your scheduled exercise appointment. Create a routine you can't live without. Your ability to be a happy, healthy, productive individual depends on it. I know it's difficult. Don't worry. I'll have more options for you later.

It Doesn't Have to Hurt

Remember the good ole days when the adage "No pain—no gain" was popular? I was raised with that school of thought. I learned it in my years of physical therapy practice, in my figure skating and martial arts life, and in the school of hard knocks. I was a pain junky! As a Marine friend used to say, *"Pain is good, extreme pain is extremely good."* Well, now I'm here to tell you that it's a load of crap! This kind of thinking is responsible for more injuries, failed diets, and aversion to exercise than any of the million excuses we can come up with not to take care of ourselves.

In all fairness, living a healthy lifestyle is no walk in the park (pardon the pun), but it doesn't have to be punishing either. Deprivation, lack of true motivation, and physical discomfort are recipes for avoidance. If you believe you have to "hurt" or feel pain to benefit from exercise, I guarantee you won't be looking forward to it. Yes, exercise should be hard work and you'll need to exert yourself to see changes in weight or fitness level, but if, after an exercise routine, you can't climb stairs, get up off the toilet seat, or brush your teeth without your muscles squealing the next day, you've clearly done too much. If you experience sharp shooting pains, numbness or tingling, or become so winded you can't hold a conversation though your workout, you need to back off and modify your program. Get rid of that *"all or none"* thinking and adopt a new message.

"Some is better than none. More is not better."

Understanding the difference between "pain" and "muscle burn" is essential for developing and maintaining a safe, effective exercise routine. First off, you need to work within a pain-free range of motion. Don't push past pain. Find the edge of what's enough and what's too much and stay on the "just enough" side. This is your "edge." It's the place where you feel your muscles working, but the sensation you feel is tolerable, and you can perform the exercise without holding your breath or gritting your teeth. Knowing where your "edge" is will help you decide where your weaknesses lie and what types of exercise are right for you.

For instance, I know that running, swimming, and biking are not for me. Not that I'm not good at any of those things or that they aren't good for me in theory, but running has repeatedly led to joint problems for me in the past, swimming requires more repetitive rotation than my unstable spine enjoys, and biking puts me in too much forward flexion, further tightening my hip flexors, hamstrings, and cervical extensors—areas of my body which are already overly tight. I've found that variety—also known as Cross Training—is the key for me. I rotate through various routines for upper and lower body resistive training, focus on core stabilization exercises, avoid repetitive or one sided sports (like tennis, bowling, and golf), and add in recreational activities that I find enjoyable and challenging, such as kayaking, hiking, or roller blading.

NOTE: The trick is to find activities you'll enjoy, stick with, and are willing to sweat through for 30 minutes five times per week.

Accept the fact that exercise needs to be a part of your life if you want to stick around and see your grandkids graduate college, or if you want to dance at your parents' seventy-fifth wedding anniversary. Of course, there are no guarantees. You could do everything right and life might still throw you a cancer curve ball or other health challenge, but fitness is a way of life that has numerous benefits and no downside if you do it right and stay on top of it. If you are lamenting your "poor quality of life," consistent exercise is #1 on the list of likely fixes.

Another suggestion for achieving success is to "buddy up." Being held accountable to a workout partner will often motivate you to get off the couch if you know you'll be "letting down" your partner. This is one of the reasons Weight Watchers is so successful. They employ partnering strategies that help you feel supported and less alone on your journey. Setting exercise goals that are manageable, measurable, and attainable, and sharing them with others will give you that push to stick with it. Let's face it, no one wants to eat crow or admit they've fallen off the wagon.

Even online support groups can be great resources. A Facebook group like Romance Fit Club for Readers and Writers, headed up by bestselling author, Sara Humphries is a priceless find. She has daily check-ins, occasionally shares her own struggles, and does all she can to offer great suggestions and advice for sticking with your program. I joined the group just for the comradery, and I find it especially inspiring on days when I'd rather be sleeping in or have to spend my entire day catching up on e-mails and word count goals. It reminds me that I can do ANYTHING for 30 minutes and that my health is the single most important factor in assuring my quality of life. I'm also reminded that I'm not alone in my struggles and that I'm always only 30 minutes away from a good mood. Don't ruin it with the "all or nothing" philosophy or the idea that you have to be "dying" to get any benefit from exercise.

In the next chapter, I'll offer basic, gentle stretches you can do anytime, anywhere. I encourage you to master them and incorporate them into your daily life.

CHAPTER 10

STRETCHING EXERCISES

The following are specific exercises you can do to help maintain flexibility, gain strength, and preserve your functional **activities of daily living** (ADLs). It really doesn't have to be a full time job, but you do need to pay attention to your body and move it in all kinds of ways to keep it functioning optimally. There is much debate on the benefits of static stretching verses dynamic stretching, but the latest research shows that dynamic stretching (stretching with movement) is best before an actual workout, and static stretching works best for the cool down phase at the end. For the purposes of this book and to simplify your life, I'll assume that most of you are not going to be doing these stretches and then going out to run a marathon. If you are, check with your trainer for more dynamic stretches that will prepare you for the event. Examples of dynamic stretching are arm circles, toe touches, or walking lunges. A stretch is considered static when you lean into it, find your edge, and hold it for a period of time. NEVER stretch beyond your comfort level or "bounce" into it. Think:

"**Stretch, hold, breathe, stretch a little further.**"

NOTE: It's not recommended to stretch "cold" muscles, so do a few minutes of warm-up to get your blood moving to your muscles before you stretch. Something as simple as marching in place and pumping your arms for a few minutes will do.

Now that we've made the proper distinctions and given you a few guidelines, let's begin with lower extremity stretches and work our way upward. After all, the feet are the base from which all other things stand.

NOTE about healthy feet: Taking care of our feet is a no brainer. They do so much for us each day, we owe them a little respect. Wear good footwear, avoid heels as much as possible, and have your feet evaluated for orthotics. You'd be amazed at how standing on the proper supportive surface can affect your knees, hips, and spine. Proper alignment starts at your feet. Make sure you show them some love.

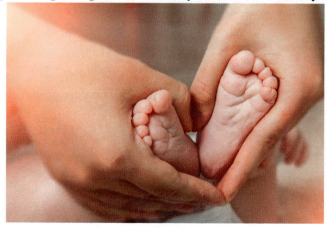

Fig. 9

Calf stretch

WHY IT'S IMPORTANT: As we age, and when we spend a lot of time sitting, the calf muscles shorten. One consequence of this is that we lose our proper heel/toe function during walking, giving us a shuffling gait, which disrupts our balance, and is a contributing factor in falls. Because of the tendon and fascial connections, tight calves also put added tension on the hamstrings and "back of the body muscles" all the way up to the neck.

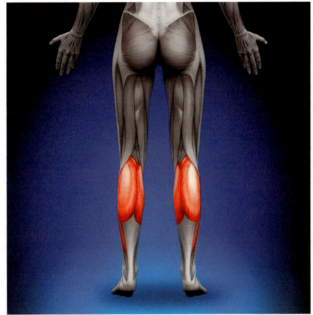

Fig. 10 Gastrocnemius (Calf Muscles)

As I pointed out earlier, our insides are covered in a web of fascia that connects to every part of our body. If your calves are tight, it can ultimately cause neck pain and even headaches. Eastern Medicine teaches that the bladder meridian runs the full length of the back of the body and the points along the calf directly relate to points in the neck. I've had firsthand relief of my neck pain from massaging the tender points along the bladder meridian on my calf.

Calf stretching will also improve circulation and help avoid clots, which can easily form with prolonged sitting. Stretching your calves can be done anywhere. The grocery store while pushing your carriage, the lunch line at work, or up against a filing cabinet or door while you're on that fifteen minute break. Instead of checking your twitter feed or Facebook page, do a few stretches and take some deep breaths. I do my calf stretches in the shower, with the lovely added benefit of the warm water easing muscle tension. Wherever you do it, make it part of your daily routine.

INSTRUCTIONS: Stand with your hands against a wall or supportive surface. Place one foot forward and one foot back and keep your toes on both feet facing straight ahead. Bend the front knee and keep the back leg straight, making sure your front knee doesn't extend out beyond your toes and that your back heel stays down. You should feel a strong stretch in your calf muscle (gastrocnemius). Be sure to stand up straight and keep your head and shoulders over your hips. Relax your shoulders and take a breath or two. Then switch sides.

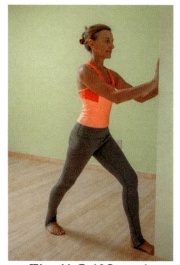

Fig. 11 Calf Stretch

NOTE: If you have balance issues, be sure to have handrails installed in your shower. Do NOT do exercises in the shower if you're prone to dizziness or have health issues requiring narcotic medications.

Hamstring Stretch

WHY IT'S IMPORTANT: Your hamstrings attach distally (below your knee), crossing the attachments to the gastrocnemius (main calf muscle), and proximally at the ischial tuberosity (the butt bones, or "sit" bones as they're called in yoga).

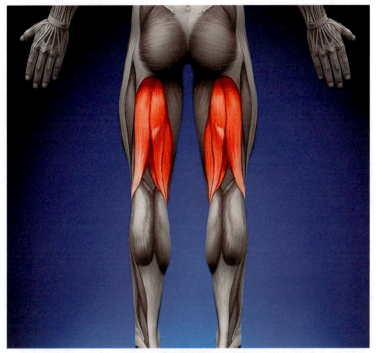

Fig. 12 Hamstrings

Tight hamstrings can cause major low back problems. When we sit too much, the hamstrings in the back of the legs and hip flexors in the front of the body (we'll be getting to those soon) shorten and become tight, causing a torqueing of the pelvis.

In other words, our hamstrings and hip flexors are at war, and the pelvis and low back are the casualties. These opposing forces cause strain and muscle imbalances, which can cause malalignment issues. This is where a chiropractor, physical therapist, massage therapist, or osteopath can come in handy. But whoever you see for treatment will have an uphill battle keeping you aligned if you aren't consistently stretching out these muscle groups to combat the poor habits that created the problem in the first place.

The hamstrings can be stretched a number of ways. I do them lying on my back in bed before I get up. It makes a remarkable difference in my ability to stand up straight and move without pain first thing in the morning. I also stretch the piriformis, which I'll show you further on.

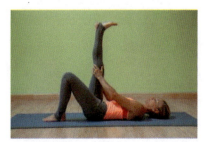

Fig. 13 Supine Hamstring Stretch

INSTRUCTIONS: Lying on your back with your feet flat. Raise one leg toward the ceiling and gently straighten the knee **(It's acceptable to hold behind your knee or thigh for support. Some people use a bathrobe tie or towel to hold the leg up).** Gently draw your toes toward your face, pressing the heel toward the ceiling. This is called dorsi-flexion. Pointing your toes would be called plantar flexion. You can add some ankle circles in each direction here to really stretch out the whole lower leg and promote circulation. Hold for a few breaths and switch sides. Repeat two to three times on each leg.

NOTE: You'll notice I'm not giving you specific hold times. I believe that's an individual determination. Ideally, you'd want to hold your stretches for thirty seconds and repeat them three times on each side. But these rigid constructs are a deterrent for many people who see exercise as a time suck and therefore will do nothing rather than do something if they feel forced to hold their stretches long enough to watch paint dry on the ceiling.

Instead of focusing on the numbers, focus on the breath and the sensation in the muscle. Take as many breaths in and out as it takes to feel the muscle tension ease. That might be one or two breaths for one person, or four to five for someone else. Just remember, the time you spend stretching will benefit you exponentially if you are patient and consistent. **Rushing through your stretches will not give you the desired effect and can even lead to injury. Relax, breathe, and practice mindfulness.**

More ways to stretch your hamstrings

Standing hamstring stretch

INSTRUCTIONS: Find a railing, chair, or wall to support yourself. Raise one leg onto a step or low chair, resting your heel down and lifting your toes toward your face. Lengthen through the crown of your head and gently press your chest forward, keeping your back straight and head up. The goal is NOT to reach your toes or bring your nose to your knee. With your leg straight and toes lifted (dorsi-flexed), you won't have to bend far at the hips to feel a strong pull up the back of the leg. Hold here and breathe. Switch to the other side and repeat two to three times.

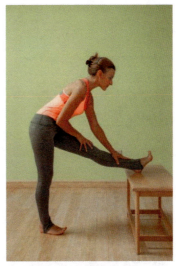

Fig. 14 Standing Hamstring Stretch

Seated hamstring stretch

INSTRUCTIONS: Sitting in a firm chair with a straight back, extend your leg. Again, dorsi-flex your foot and gently press out through your heel. The taller you can sit up straight with shoulders back and chest lifted, the more you'll feel it in the back of your leg. If needed, you can modify by scooting to the edge of your chair, resting your heel down onto the floor, and leaning forward slightly. Keep the leg straight to maximize the benefit of the stretch.

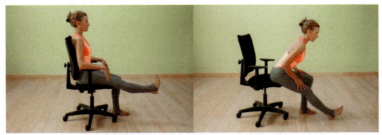

Fig. 15a Seated Hamstring Stretch   Fig. 15b Modification

Adductor (inner thigh) Stretch

WHY IT'S IMPORTANT: The muscles of the inner thigh, several of which attach below the knee and travel up to the pelvis, are often neglected in our stretching routines. Unless we ride horseback, we don't use these muscles on a regular basis for our daily activities, but if you're a runner or athlete, you know that a "groin pull" (aka, adductor strain) can sideline you for weeks or even months. With prolonged sitting, the adductors become shortened and tight, creating an increased risk of injury with simple ADLs like crossing your ankle over your knee to tie your shoe or squatting to lift something heavy.

INSTRUCTIONS: There are several excellent ways to stretch this muscle group. The gentlest way to stretch is seated in your chair, feet flat and knees spread wide with toes turned out. Place your hands on your knees and with a flat back and head up, press your chest forward until you feel a stretch on the inner thighs. Gently press outward on the knees to deepen the stretch. (Not shown.)

Another option is to sit on the floor/mat, bring the soles of your feet together and gently press your knees down toward the floor. Don't force the stretch. Allow the knees and hips to open gently.

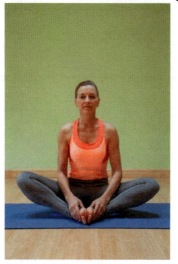

Fig. 16 Butterfly Stretch

A third option and one for more advanced stretching, is to do a wide angle forward fold, either in sitting or standing. In sitting, bring legs apart to a comfortable wide angle with toes lifted. You can stay here and simply work on sitting up straight until you feel comfortable enough to walk your hands forward. Keep your spine long and chest lifted. If this is difficult, you can lean against a wall and place small towel rolls under your knees until your flexibility increases.

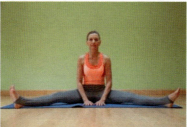

Fig. 17 Wide Angle Forward Fold

To focus the stretch on one leg at a time, slowly reach for the toes (or the knee or ankle depending on your flexibility) on one side. I'll repeat here that **quality of movement is more important than quantity of movement**. As always, listen to your body and respect your limitations. Hold the stretch for three to five breaths and repeat two to three times on each side.

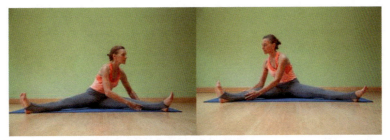

Fig. 18a Reach Toward Left   Fig. 18b Reach Toward Right

Quadriceps stretch

WHY IT'S IMPORTANT: The quadriceps, or front of the thigh muscles, are a group of four muscles which attach distally (below the knee at the bony prominence called the tibial tuberosity), and proximally at the pelvis and around the hip joint. This massive group of muscles is responsible for straightening the knee, raising the leg, and pretty much every movement required for locomotion. These powerhouse muscles are needed for everything from walking and stair climbing to jumping and kicking—and everything in between. Since the attachments are closely related anatomically to the hip flexor muscles, the quads also tend to get tight and weak with prolonged sitting and should be stretched daily to reduce stress on the lower back. You'll see why when we talk about the hip flexors, also shown below.

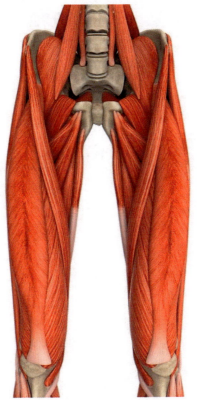

Fig. 19 Quadriceps, hip flexors, and deep hip musculature

INSTRUCTIONS: Standing, hold onto a firm/stationary surface, bend your knee up toward your chest until you can reach your ankle or foot behind you. Clasping the ankle/foot, lower the knee so it points down toward the floor and pull the heel in toward the glutes. Keep your belly tuned in and tuck your tailbone slightly downward to increase the stretch and avoid arching the back. Try to keep the knee pointing down toward the floor and avoid pulling the foot outward away from the body. If you find that you don't have the flexibility to do this without twisting your back, getting a hamstring cramp, or otherwise struggling to maintain good alignment, move to plan B or C as needed.

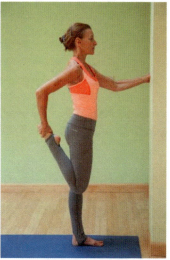

Fig. 20a Standing Quadricep Stretch

Plan B: Holding on to a firm/stationary surface, swing your foot up and around onto a chair behind you so that the top of your foot/shin rests on the seat with your knee pointing downward and your hips facing straight ahead. You should feel a stretch up the front of your thigh. Add height to the chair seat by propping pillows up until you feel as if you have a good stretch or are able to progress to holding onto your foot or ankle.

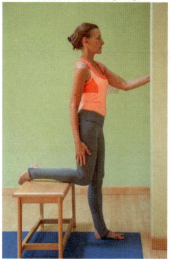

Fig. 20b Modified Quadricep Stretch

Plan C: If standing quad stretches are still too difficult or you find yourself struggling to hold the stretch, try it in side lying as shown below. You can use a belt or strap wrapped around the ankle and pull it in toward your glutes if you can't reach your foot comfortably or have limited range of motion at the knee joint. Do whatever you need to do to make it work while focusing on good alignment and breathing.

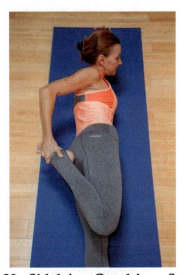

Fig. 20c Sidelying Quadricep Stretch

NOTE: This stretch should be felt in the thigh, **NOT** the knee. If you have decreased ROM and can't do this stretch without knee pain, skip it or see a physical therapist or personal trainer for other options.

Hip flexor stretch

WHY IT'S IMPORTANT: The hip flexor muscles (made up of the psoas major and minor, and the iliacus) are located in the front of your hip. They attach distally onto the femur (thigh bone) and proximally along the lumbar vertebrae and even into the twelfth thoracic vertebrae. It's difficult to conceptualize the complexity and importance of this muscle group without understanding exactly where the muscles attach and how they work. The action of the hip flexor group is to raise your leg to the front, such as with marching, or even stepping up a stair or lifting your leg to tie your shoe. These muscles run through your pelvis and attach into your lower back and are a major contributor to low back pain when they become tight or weak, both of which happen with prolonged sitting.

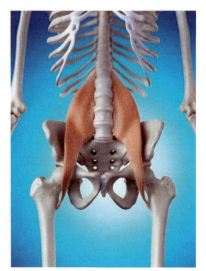 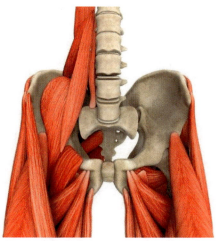

Fig. 21 Psoas Major (hip flexor)   Fig. 22 Hip Flexor Complex

INSTRUCTIONS: Again, if balance is an issue for you, find something sturdy to hold onto while doing these standing stretches. I'd rather have you focus on correct form than flopping all over the place trying not to fall. Take a large step forward and bend your front knee. Remember to observe the knee over the ankle alignment here so you aren't stressing your front knee. The back leg should be far enough behind you so that you are on the ball of the foot with heel raised and you can extend out through the sole of the foot. Tilt your pelvis slightly by contracting your abdominals and tucking your tailbone downward. This should "turn on" the stretch in the front of the back leg and hip. If you still aren't feeling it, bend deeper into the front knee and lift up through your crown, shoulders back and down. Hold for several breaths and switch sides. Repeat two to three times each side.

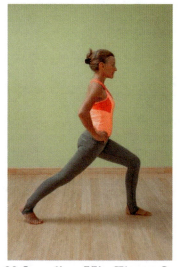

Fig. 23 Standing Hip Flexor Stretch

Seated hip flexor stretch

INSTRUCTIONS: If you find the standing version too challenging or need to stretch this muscle while in the midst of a meeting, you can do so in sitting. Turn sideways in your chair as shown below. Holding onto the arm of the chair for support, and keeping one side of your glutes fully connected to the chair, place your front foot solidly on the ground with knee over ankle. Now stretch your back leg straight out behind you, lifting the heel off the ground and pressing out through the sole of the foot as above. If you don't feel much stretch, engage your pelvic tuck and lift up tall through your spine, shoulders down, chest lifted. Feel free to get the whole board room doing it!

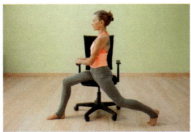

Fig. 24 Seated Hip Flexor Stretch

Standing Back Extension

Whenever you've been sitting for any length of time, either at your desk, in a movie theatre, or in your car, this next stretch should be employed. You probably do this one naturally, just because it feels good and your body WANTS it.

CAUTION: Avoid extension exercises if you have spinal stenosis and discontinue if the exercise aggravates your pain symptoms or increases lower extremity radiculopathy (symptoms down the leg).

INSTRUCTIONS: Stand up from your chair, place your hands on your hips, and bring your feet hip width apart. Keep your knees slightly bent and your chin tucked down to avoid straining your neck. Now, lift up through your chest and lengthen your spine before gently arching backwards while pressing your hips forward. This modified "back bend" will not only stretch your hip flexors and abdominals, it will stretch your pectoral muscles which attach in the chest and front of the shoulders, two areas that get super tight with prolonged sitting. We'll talk about specific stretches for these muscle groups coming up.

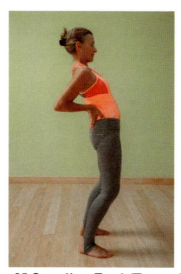

Fig. 25 Standing Back Extension

Piriformis stretch (hip rotator)

WHY IT'S IMPORTANT: The piriformis attaches distally at the greater trochanter of the femur and proximally at the medial border of the sacrum. It is not only an external rotator of the hip, it is one of the primary stabilizers of the sacrum and pelvis. With prolonged sitting, this muscle becomes overstretched and weak, which leads to tightness and muscle imbalances that can easily cause sacral malalignment issues. This muscle is often responsible for the proverbial "pain in the butt." In some cases, the sciatic nerve runs through this muscle and tightness or spasm here can cause lower extremity pain, numbness and/or tingling, aka, sciatica. Read more about this in the **TREATMENT** section.

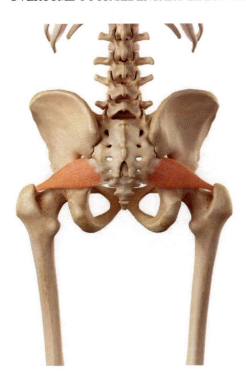

Fig. 26 Piriformis

INSTRUCTIONS: There are several ways to stretch the piriformis and gluteal muscles. I'll give you my "before jumping out of bed" version first. Lying on your back with knees bent and feet flat, cross your ankle over the opposite knee and then drop your knees to that side (for instance, if you are crossing your right ankle over the left knee, drop your knees to the left). Arms will be stretched out in a T position and your head will be turned to the right so you get a spinal twist from tail to head. If this is too much, you can support your knees on a pillow or with your hand. Hold each stretch for two to three breaths and repeat two to three times on each side.

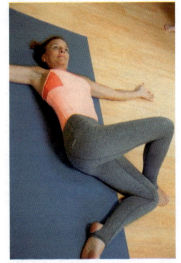

Fig. 27a Piriformis, ITB, and Low Back Stretch

If you need a modification because your lower back lacks flexibility, try one of these.

b) Knees bent, feet flat, cross your left ankle over your right knee and gently pull it in toward your opposite shoulder.

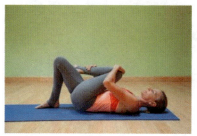

Fig. 27b Simple Piriformis Stretch

c) Figure four stretch-Cross right ankle over left knee, reach between your thighs and wrap your hands around the back of your left leg. Pull your knees in toward your chest.

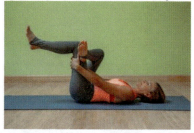

Fig 27c Figure Four Piriformis Stretch

Sitting Piriformis Stretch

INSTRUCTIONS: Seated in a firm, straight-backed chair, cross your left ankle over your right knee. Lift up through the crown of your head, lean slightly forward, keeping your back straight. You should feel a stretch in the left gluteal muscles and high hamstring. Stay and breathe for two to three breaths and then switch sides. Repeat two to three times on each side.

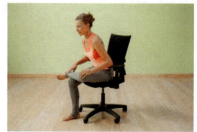

Fig. 28 Seated Piriformis Stretch

Standing Piriformis Stretch

INSTRUCTIONS: Holding on to a firm/stationary object like a door frame or countertop, shift your weight onto your right leg and bend your knee. Cross your left ankle above your right knee and sit back, gently pressing your hips out behind you as if reaching to sit in a chair. It's important to keep the back straight, chest lifted, and spine long, as well as hinging at the hips to engage the piriformis muscle in the stretch. Sink as low as is comfortable or until you feel the stretch into the right gluteal muscles. **NOTE: Avoid bending the standing knee out past the toes as this will strain the knee. If you feel stress in the knee, sit back further with the hips or come up on the knee until proper alignment is achieved.** Hold for two to three breaths and switch sides. Repeat two to three times each side.

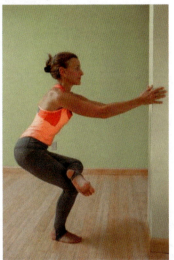

Fig. 29 Standing Piriformis Stretch

ADVANCED Hip Flexor and Piriformis stretches

If you already practice yoga on a regular basis or are fairly fit, you may be familiar with these two poses (asanas) and find these advanced moves the perfect way to get into those hard to reach places like the iliacus, oblique abdominals, and deep hip rotators like the piriformis.

When in doubt, please be sensible and realistic about your fitness level, and don't try these at home without some one-on-one instruction from your yoga teacher or personal trainer.

Pigeon Pose (Eka Pada Rajakapotasana)

I know that's a mouthful, isn't it? It's not so important that you know the Sanskrit name for this fabulous hip opening yoga pose, but it is important that you be well warmed up before attempting it. I also encourage students to use bolstering as needed to get comfortable in this pose. Have a firm pillow, rolled blanket, or yoga block nearby to tuck under your front hip if it feels like too much of a stretch or your hip doesn't reach the floor. Pigeon pose is great for not only stretching the hip flexors on the back leg, but the piriformis and deep hip rotators on the front leg.

INSTRUCTIONS: Begin on all fours in "table" position. Extend one leg out behind you and then slide it forward until your knee rests between your hands and the heel rests in front of the hip of the back leg. Here is where you can place a block or other support under your buttock if you can't easily get it down to the floor. The illustrations below show views from both sides so you can see foot and bolster placement.

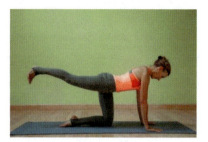

Fig. 30 Hip Extension in Table

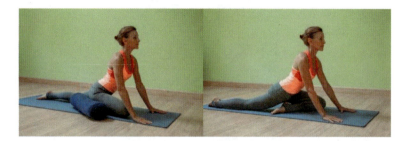

Fig. 31a Pidgeon w/Bolster Under Hip   Fig. 31b Pidgeon Pose

From here, work the back leg a little further behind you so you can feel the stretch into the hip flexors on that leg. To deepen further, curl your toes under, lift the knee slightly and press out through the heel. As always, lift up through the crown, lengthen the spine and relax your shoulders down and back. Breathe! If you are very flexible and comfortable here, you can also rest forward onto your forearms or forehead and hang out there for a few breaths in a posture known as King Pigeon.

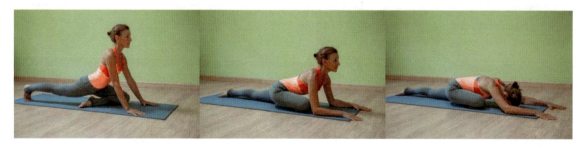

Fig. 31c   Fig. 31d   Fig. 31e

More ADVANCED—Downward facing dog (Adho Mukha Svanasana) (3 legged version with torso rotation)

Yikes, you say! If this looks intimidating, feel free to skip it. There's no one watching over your shoulder, and yoga is not about striving or pushing yourself into uncomfortable positions. However, if you have a yoga practice and can manage a steady downward facing dog pose, this little "extra" can hit you in all the right places.

INSTRUCTIONS: Begin in table (on hands and knees). Set your palms out in front of you at shoulder width apart. Make sure your palms are connected to the mat with fingers spread wide and the middle finger pointing forward. Curl your toes under, lift your tail skyward, and press your hips up toward the ceiling, creating a triangle shape with your body.

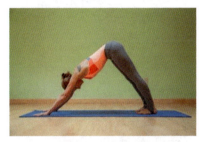

Fig. 32 Downward facing Dog

It's okay to have your knees bent if you aren't flexible enough yet. Gently work towards straightening your knees and lowering your heels toward the mat before moving on to the next step. Come in and out of this pose as needed until you can hold it with relative ease and breathe comfortably. Feel free to rest in Child's pose in between tries. (See Child's Pose Below).

NOTE: It takes time to condition the body to tolerate these deeper stretches. That's why Yoga is called a practice. It may take many weeks—even months—before downward dog is mastered. Stay with it until you can hold the pose for five breaths before moving on to the next level.

Next, center your left foot on the mat and lift your right leg out and up behind you. Lengthen out through the leg without rotating the hips just yet. Once you have a strong, balanced single leg stance, bend your right heel in toward your left glute, keeping the hips level.

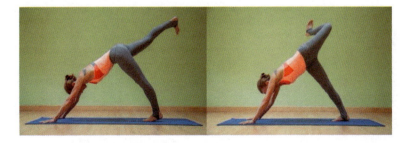

Fig. 32a Three Legged Dog   Fig. 32b Broken-Legged Dog

Once you have good balance there, begin to open your left hip by rotating the pelvis. Extend the leg, point the toe, and look up at your right hand. You'll feel a nice stretch through the iliacus and oblique muscles of the abdomen as well as in your lats, the large upper back muscle that connects from your arm to your lower back. Stay and breathe a few breaths and then reverse the motion to come back to table.

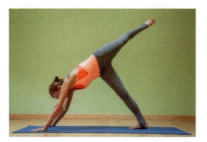

Fig. 32c Three Legged Dog w/ Hip Opener

It's always nice to sink into Child's Pose and relax here for a few breaths before moving on to the other side. Rest your hands at your heels to give your shoulders some relief.

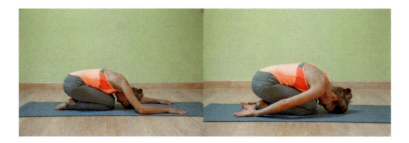

Fig 33a Child's Pose   **Fig. 33b Simple Child**

BONUS: If you're feeling adventurous or want to combine movements to create a short Vinyasa flow after mastering the individual postures, go from Downward Facing Dog (DFD) to Pigeon by looking up toward your hands and sliding your knee up between them. Settle into Pigeon pose, stay and breathe for a few breaths, and then curl your toes under and slide the front foot back to meet the right. Hold in plank before pushing back up into DFD. Repeat on the other side before coming to rest in Child's pose. I've been known to hold a minute long Plank pose in between DFD and Pigeon. We'll talk more about Planks soon.

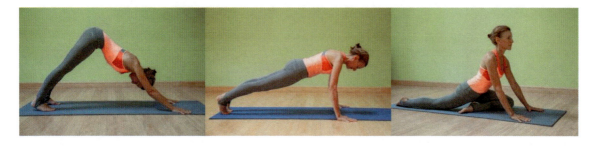

Fig. 34 DFD   **Fig. 35 Plank**   **Fig. 31b Pidgeon**

Gentle Lower Back stretches

WHY IT'S IMPORTANT: The lower back, along with the abdominals, comprise our core. (For now I'll leave out the scapular stabilizers and upper torso musculature, which I also consider core musculature.) Sitting causes our abdominals to shorten and become week, while our lower back is in a tug of war with our tight hip flexors. It's no wonder, by day's end, we're feeling achy and exhausted.

The natural curve of the lumbar spine is seriously compromised with prolonged sitting. Our vertebrae, sacrum, pelvis and coccyx were not designed for static compressive forces, which, over time, cause maladaptive imbalances, wear and tear on the joints, and reduced disc spaces. **Stretching and strengthening can help!**

Knee to Chest Stretch

I'm sure you're all familiar with most of these stretches, but proper instruction is always a good idea, and a refresher never hurts.

INSTRUCTIONS: Lie on your back with knees bent and feet flat. Draw one knee into your chest and then the other. You can choose to do these one at a time, hold for a few breaths, and alternate them, or draw both in at the same time for a bilateral lower back stretch. **Be sure to relax your shoulders, neck, and face.** Stretching shouldn't involve a lot of effort, and the benefits are far reaching if you focus on your breath and relax. Take this time to reflect on something you're grateful for. It makes the time pass and gives you a spiritual boost. *Put on the garment of praise for the spirit of heaviness.* Isaiah 61:3 Better advice was never given. Gratitude always pulls me out of the mire of negative thinking.

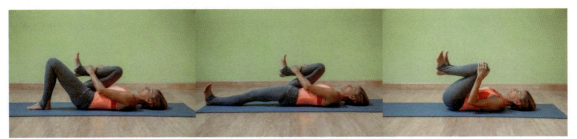

Fig. 36a Single Knee to Chest   Fig. 36b SKC w/Hip Flexor Stretch   Fig. 36c Double Knee to Chest

Alternatively, you can extend one leg down to the floor and press out through the heel as you gently tighten your thigh. This should add a stretch to the hip flexors and calf muscles of the extended leg. Contract your abdominals by drawing your belly button in toward your spine and gently pressing your lower back into the mat. This is called a pelvic tilt and will be a staple part of our routine once we reach the strengthening phase.

Knee Rocks Side to Side (Lower Trunk Rotation)

Lie on your back with knees bent feet flat. Bring your arms out to the sides in a T position. Let your knees fall to one side while looking over the opposite shoulder. This should give you a gentle spinal twist. Hold and breathe, then repeat on the other side. It helps protect your back if you engage your abdominals when bringing your knees back to center.

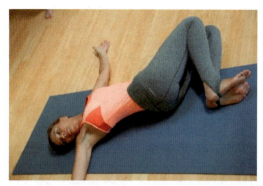

Fig. 37 Lower Trunk Rotation (Knee Rocks Side to Side)

ADVANCED: I gave you this one earlier as a piriformis stretch, but it's my go to morning stretch for opening the lower back and hip. Cross your right ankle over your left knee. Drop your knees to the left. Hold for two to three breaths. Come back to center and switch sides. This gets deeper into the low back and also stretches the piriformis and ITB. The ITB or **iliotibial band**, is a wide band of connective tissue that runs from the iliac crest (hip bone), along the outer thigh, and attaches at the lateral knee. Tightness of the ITB is one of the main culprits for hip bursitis and knee pain.

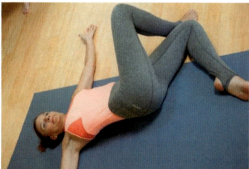

Fig. 27a Piriformis, ITB, and Low Back Stretch

MORE ADVANCED: For an extra stretch to the ITB, slowly straighten your top leg and point your toes down toward the floor. Feel free to use your hand to support the leg and control how deeply you stretch. Avoid this one if you have low back instability, nerve pain, or lack the flexibility to do this comfortably. Use props such as a pillow or block under the leg for support as needed.

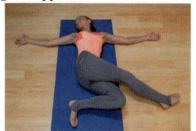

Fig. 38 Advanced ITB Stretch

Seated Low Back Stretch (Seated Forward Fold)

This one is for desk dwellers who need a quick fix to hold them over between *real* stretch breaks.

INSTRUCTIONS: Sit with your feet slightly wider than hip width apart and planted on the floor. Slowly fold forward, allowing your hands to slide down the inner thigh and lower leg until you reach the floor (or ankles or shins, depending upon your flexibility). Hang in this forward fold, relaxing your neck and gently stretching the lower back. Take a few deep breaths. Slowly rise up by tucking your belly button into your spine and rolling up as if stacking your vertebrae one on top of the other. **NOTE: If you have lower back issues and find this difficult, you can rest your elbows/forearms on your knees for support.**

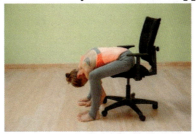

Fig. 39 Seated Forward Fold

Seated Trunk Rotation

INSTRUCTIONS: Sitting up straight with your feet flat on the floor and hip width apart, reach the right hand to the left knee and the left arm around the back of the chair. Lift up through the crown of the head and look over the left shoulder as if trying to bring your belly button toward your left hip. Hold and breathe, and repeat on the other side, coming back to center between each rotation. For a deeper stretch into the hip and piriformis, cross the left leg over the right. Repeat two to three times on each side.

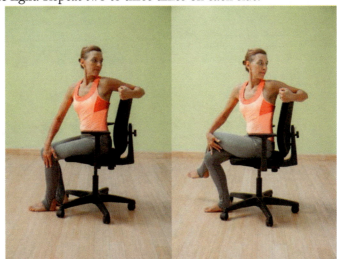

Fig. 40a Trunk Rotation Stretch   Fig. 40b Trunk Rotation w/Piriformis Stretch

Seated Side Bending

INSTRUCTIONS: Sitting with your feet flat and a little wider than hip width apart, reach your left hand down the side of the chair toward the floor. At the same time, reach your right hand up toward the ceiling, extending out through the fingertips. Keep your sits bones connected to the chair and try not to collapse into the stretch. Imagine keeping both sides of the spine long as you side bend and reach. Hold and breathe, and repeat on each side two to three times.

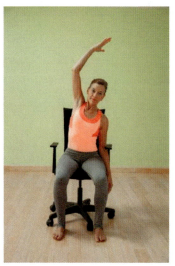

Fig. 41 Seated Side Bending Stretch

Upper Back Stretch (Arm pulls across front of body) (Rhomboid and mid traps stretch)

INSTRUCTIONS: Sitting or standing up straight, reach across your body with your left arm. Clasp your left wrist with your right hand. Relax the shoulder away from the ear and gently pull arm across the body to the right. You can add a rotation of the head to the left (not shown) to increase the stretch. Hold and breathe, and repeat two to three times on each side.

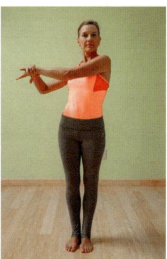

Fig. 42 Rhomboid (Upper Back) Stretch

Triceps Stretch with Lateral Side Bend (Triceps and latissimus)

INSTRUCTIONS: Sitting or standing up straight, raise your left arm overhead and reach down toward the center of your back as if to scratch an itch between your shoulder blades. With your right hand, gently press the left elbow up toward the ceiling and slightly back. You'll feel a strong stretch in the back of the upper arm. Add a slight side bend to the right to move the stretch deeper into the upper back and shoulder, applying the stretch to the latissimus dorsi muscle or lats.

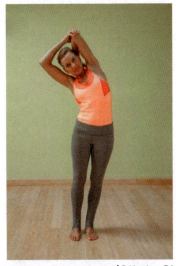

Fig. 43 Triceps Stretch w/Slight Side Bend

Biceps and Chest Stretch (Biceps, anterior deltoid, and pectoralis muscles)

INSTRUCTIONS: Sitting or standing up straight, bring both hands directly in front of you at shoulder height with palms turned up. Extend your arms out to the side and back as if serving bowls of soup to the people behind you. Hold and breathe. Then lower your arms to half way (45 degree angle out from the body), and turn the palms down and back, stretching a little deeper into the shoulder (not shown).

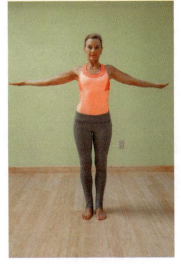

Fig. 44 Bicep Stretch

Alternatively, you can stretch your pecs by clasping your hands behind your back and pressing your knuckles down toward your heels as you squeeze your shoulder blades together. This won't stretch the biceps specifically, but it is an excellent shoulder and chest opener.

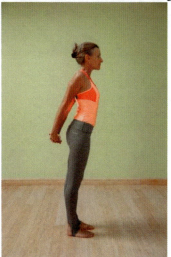

Fig. 45 Pectoralis Stretch

Wrist Flexor and Extensor Stretches

WHY IT'S IMPORTANT: These wrist stretches are an essential part of your arsenal for staving off Carpal Tunnel Syndrome and many other hand/wrist disorders caused from repetitive strain and overuse. Adding these alone can make a huge difference!

INSTRUCTIONS: Extend your arm out in front of you at a ninety degree angle with your palm facing down. **NOTE: It's important to have the elbow completely straight to get the most benefit from the stretch.** Raise your fingertips toward the ceiling, and with the opposite hand, gently pull back on your fingers until you feel a stretch along the underside of your forearm, stretching the wrist flexor muscles.

Alternatively, you can turn the palm up and stretch the fingers downward for a deeper stretch to the flexors, adding a nice bonus stretch to the pronator muscles of the forearm and a bicep stretch. Hold and breathe, switch sides and repeat on the opposite hand. Repeat the exercise two to three times and include it often throughout your workday stretch breaks.

OVERCOME YOUR SEDENTARY LIFESTYLE

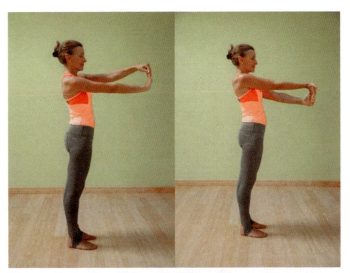

Fig. 46a Wrist Flexor Stretch   Fig. 46b Wrist Flexor, Pronator, and Biceps Stretch

To stretch the topside of the forearm—the wrist extensors—simply reverse the motion, beginning with the palm face down and pointing the fingertips downward. With the opposite hand, gently pull the fingers down and toward you. Hold two to three breaths and repeat two to three times on each side.

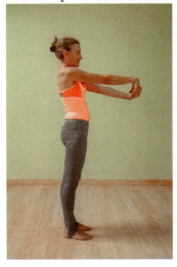

Fig. 47 Wrist Extensor Stretches

CAUTION: Don't force the stretch. Be gentle and only apply the amount of pressure needed to feel the stretch up the arm into the muscles. If you don't feel a stretch and you've been having wrist pain or elbow tendonitis issues, you might consider wrist braces to offer support for your strained muscles and unstable joints. See more in the **TREATMENT** section.

Neck Stretches

WHY IT'S IMPORTANT: The cervical spine is made up of a complex series of gliding joints which work together with the muscles to forward flex, extend, rotate, and side bend the seven cervical vertebrae that top off the spine and support the cranium. The slight curve and upward angle of the bones creates the perfect biomechanical advantage for holding the head in alignment over the rest of the spine and allows for a unique combination of movements, giving us optimal range of motion.

Remember that ten to twelve pound head we all carry on our shoulders? I believe I used the illustration of holding a ten pound bowling ball in close to your body. It won't weigh that much, but try holding it out in front of you for a while. It will quickly get heavy. In fact, for every inch that you allow your head to jut out in front of your shoulders, you are adding an additional ten pounds to the weight of your head. That means that if your head is three inches out in front of your shoulders—a feat easily accomplished by most desk dwellers—your head weighs thirty pounds. Yikes! Those poor neck muscles. No wonder they're working so hard.

With the typical forward head posture inherent with prolonged sitting, the posterior muscles become tight and the anterior muscles become weak. These tight cervical muscles, which attach at the base of the skull, can contribute to headaches and even migraines because they often cut off blood supply or pinch off nerves going to and from the brain. If you sometimes get a stabbing pain that shoots over the top of your head and lands just behind your eye in a vicious throb, there's a good chance that a tight muscle pinching the ocular nerve is causing it. The stretches in this book can help. Obviously, if the pain is severe or persistent, or is worsened by stretching, seek medical care immediately. I'll give you a specific treatment protocol later on in the chapter on **TREATMENT**.

Restoring muscle balance and appropriate strength of cervical musculature is essential in helping you fight off the ravages of SLS.

Basic Cervical Range of Motion

INSTRUCTION: This is an easy one and can be done anywhere and everywhere. Sit or stand up tall, turn your head to look as far to the left as you can without pain. Hold for a breath, come back to center, and then look to the other side. Now slowly look down, then look up, and next, tip your ear toward your shoulder, repeating on each side. Do the entire sequence three to five times, following your breath through the movement. Avoid combining movements or doing "neck rolls" as these can wreak havoc with the joints of the cervical spine.

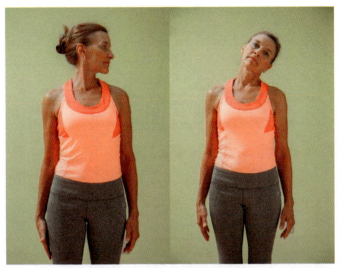

Fig. 48a Cervical Rotation   Fig. 48b Lateral Flexion (Side Bending)

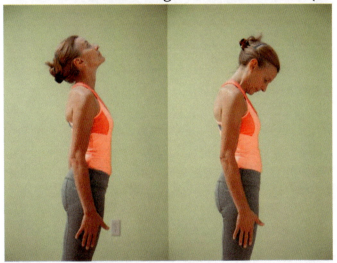

Fig. 48c Cervical Extension   Fig. 48d Cervical Flexion

NOTE: If you don't have full range of motion (ROM), just go as far as is comfortable. I'll give you a few tricks in the TREATMENT section to deal with "sticky" vertebrae.

Scalene Stretch
(Deep stabilizing muscles of the neck that are generally overworked and tight.)

INSTRUCTIONS: Tip right ear toward right shoulder and reach your left arm behind your back. You should feel a stretch into the front of your neck just above your collarbone. These are your scalene muscles. To increase the stretch, gently rest your right hand over your left ear, allowing only the weight of the hand to enhance the stretch. **DON'T pull on your head!** In fact, when you want to release the stretch, you may find it most comfortable to guide the head back to neutral using the palm of your right hand on your right cheek. Hold for three to five breaths and repeat two to three times on each side.

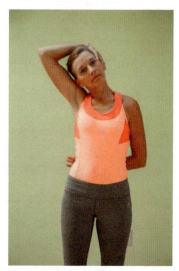

Fig. 49 Scalene Stretch

Shoulder Shrugs and Rolls

INSTRUCTIONS: This one is self-explanatory. Shrug your shoulders up and roll your shoulders backwards in a circular motion. This is a great one for releasing tension in the shoulders and neck when you've been sitting too long. A variation of this—and one I like to do frequently—is to place your fingertips on your shoulders and make circles with your elbows. This really loosens and lubricates those tight shoulder joints.

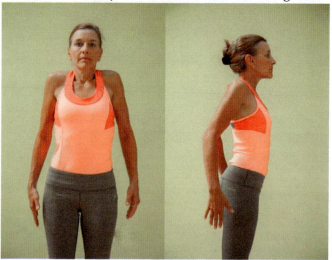

Fig. 50a Shoulder Shrugs   **Fig. 50b Shoulder Rolls**

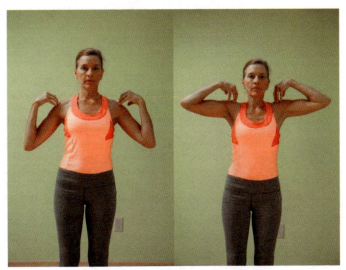

Fig. 51a and 51b Elbow Circles

NOTE regarding fascia: I can't talk about stretching of muscles without mentioning fascia. Generally, stretching alone has little effect on fascia and connective tissue unless stretches are held for up to 30-60 seconds or 5-10 breaths and repeated consistently over a long period of time. Receiving myofascial release from a massage therapist and/or acupuncture may help improve fascial pliability. Rolfing, a consistent yoga practice, craniosacral therapy, and Qi Gong seem to also have positive effects on the fascial system. Perhaps because they approach it from an energetic aspect as well as a biomechanical one. If you have struggled with Fibromyalgia, Chronic Fatigue Syndrome, or other conditions that affect the musculoskeletal system and aren't responding to other therapies, consider seeking out someone who works specifically on the fascial system or check out John Barnes's (a PT who pioneered the MFR—Myofascial Release—treatment approach) website to find a therapist in your area. http://myofascialrelease.com/

Final Note on Stretching: There are many ways to stretch each muscle and I've only given you a few. Try to do them all daily, but feel free to spread them out. I do my knee to chest stretches, knee rocks side to side, as well as hamstring and piriformis stretching before I get out of bed, and sometimes again when I lie down at night. I stretch my calves, quads, hip flexors, and hamstrings in the shower and practice Mountain pose with five to ten breaths while I'm there. I've been known to stretch in airports and lines, standing at the back of the movie theatre halfway through a two hour flick, and I have a whole car stretching routine I can do on my way to the office. Incorporating stretching into your life takes mindfulness and intention, but it's totally worth it!

Now that your muscles are longer and you've worked out some of the kinks, let's talk about strengthening.

CHAPTER 11

STRENGTHENING EXERCISES

I hope you found the stretching section helpful and user friendly. Flexibility is important but functional mobility also requires strength. You want to be able to carry a bag of groceries up a flight of stairs without sucking wind, and hopefully, you want to continue enjoying an active lifestyle with loved ones.

Having a strong, flexible body will see you through to your elder years and add to the longevity of your independence.

I'll start as before with lower extremity strengthening exercises and work toward the neck and upper extremities. Realize that these are only the basics. I want you to have simple tools that you can use to improve your overall health, fitness, and well-being. This book isn't an exercise book per se, but a tool chest of options you can easily incorporate into your daily routine. The following exercises touch on the major muscle groups and the stabilizers that are inherently weak in desk dwellers and are often overlooked in fitness routines.

As with all exercise, if it hurts, STOP! Listen to your body and work within your limitations. If an exercise feels too difficult or you can't perform it correctly, find ways to modify it to your fitness level by reducing range of motion or resistance. And remember, quality always trumps quantity. I'd rather you do five reps correctly than twenty-five incorrectly. **Our goal is to re-train your muscles to stabilize and support your spine** not build bulk or look like a fashion model. Not that there's anything wrong with building muscle or working toward a lean physique, but you don't need to be able to bench press a car. You do need to be able to sit up straight at your desk and climb a flight of stairs without stopping to rest. For the purposes of this book, we'll focus on functional strength and body awareness.

NOTE: When performing resistive exercises, focus on breathing in through the nose while at rest, and exhaling through the mouth (as if blowing through a straw) upon the exertion of the muscle.

The Basics of Pelvic Neutral Positioning

Finding Pelvic Neutral

INSTRUCTIONS: Lying on your back on a firm surface with your knees bent and feet flat, find ***pelvic neutral.*** **Pelvic neutral is the position between flexion and extension of your spine, where your abdominal muscles and lumbar extensors are working together to keep you stable.** Find neutral by first doing a pelvic tilt (pressing your lower back into the mat) and then arching your spine (lifting the belly button toward the ceiling). Now back away from those movements until you feel your abdominal muscles contract slightly and you are somewhere in the middle of those end ranges of motion. **This is your neutral position.** I'll be talking about this position frequently throughout the book, so be sure to master it before trying any of the following exercises. You'll want to be able to find neutral position lying down, sitting, and standing.

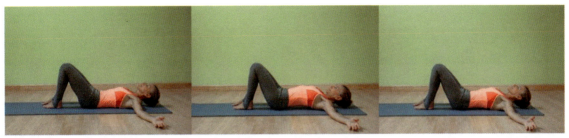

Fig. 52a Pelvic Tilt   Fig. 52b Lumbar Extension   Fig. 52c Find Pelvic Neutral

Basic Glut Sets

INSTRUCTIONS: Squeeze a pillow between your knees to engage your adductors and then squeeze your buttock muscles. (Imagine you have a hundred dollar bill between your "cheeks" and you don't want to let it go.) **NOTE: It's natural to want to do a pelvic tilt here, but our goal is to train you to maintain a neutral spine position, so avoid pressing the back down flat.** Hold for five seconds or focus on the breath for one or two cycles. Repeat ten times. Relax between reps. You can do this one in sitting, standing, or lying down. Glut sets have the added benefit of tightening the pelvic floor and can be combined with Kegel exercises (tightening up and in on the vaginal wall). This can improve the strength of the internal muscles which can assist with bladder control and sexual function. Win, win!

Dead Bugs

This seemingly simple, and what some might think silly, exercise is designed to train/strengthen your stabilizers to work together while your arms and legs are moving. Coordinated movements like these are part of everyday life and we don't want to have to think about holding neutral position when we're walking or doing our chores. We want our muscles to automatically find and hold neutral. Dead bugs are the perfect training tool and not as easy as they look. See if you can build up to doing thirty reps without any side to side movement of the hips or clicking and popping in the lower back.

INSTRUCTIONS: Lying on your back with feet flat, find neutral position. Elevate your arms overhead so the fingers are pointing up toward the ceiling. Extend your left leg out and down, stopping six inches from the floor. At the same time move your right arm down to your opposite hip and your left arm all the way over head as if you're trying to touch the floor. Don't allow your back to arch. Bring the arms and legs back to start and repeat on the other side. When you've mastered the move and can do it thirty times, try increasing the speed, but don't sacrifice quality of movement. If you lose neutral, slow down and begin again or shorten up the range of motion and don't extend your leg all the way out.

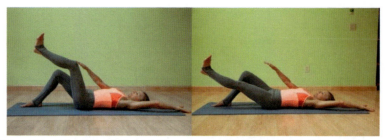

Fig. 53a Modified Dead BugFig. 53b Full Dead Bug

Bridging

INSTRUCTIONS: Now that you've trained yourself to find and maintain neutral position, you can move on to bridging. With knees bent and feet flat, press into all four corners of your feet, reach your fingertips toward your heels, gently press your arms into the mat, and lift your hips off the floor. **NOTE: This is different from bridging in yoga, where you are often encouraged to lift as high as you can and arch the back. Here, we want to maintain neutral position through the entire movement.**

Once you're in your bridge position, hold for two to three breaths and lower slowly. Repeat five to ten times. You can build up on reps and hold times as you master the move. Your goal is to eventually be able to hold a bridge position for up to three minutes. Yes, you heard that correctly. Three minutes! Set a timer or hold your bridge through a full round of commercials.

The benefits of a strong, stable back cannot be understated. If you've lived with an unstable spine that goes out of alignment frequently and derails you for days at a time, you know what I'm talking about. Mastering this move is essential. In addition to adding to the time element, you can also increase the difficulty by lifting one leg, but be sure you don't compromise your neutral position. Keep the hips level throughout the move. Work up to a five second hold time and alternate legs. Shoot for ten to twenty repetitions.

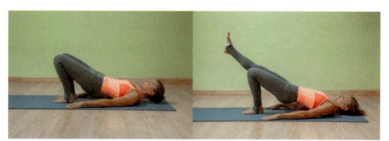

Fig. 54a BridgeFig. 54b Single Leg Bridge

More Core Stabilizing Exercises

WHY IT'S IMPORTANT: You're probably beginning to see that there is a method to my madness. I'm giving you very basic moves, but they are highly effective at retraining and strengthening your postural musculature, which is essential for minimizing the muscle imbalances your sitting career has created. Not only is it important to stretch and strengthen, but it's imperative that your muscles learn how to work together in a balanced way to support you.

Multi-joint, multi-limb activities that require coordinated muscle movements have several benefits. They force your heart to work harder to pump blood to all your moving parts, and they "train" your muscles to work together to stabilize your spine for optimal function with ADL's. You don't want your back to do all the work when you're lifting something heavy, right? We want legs, hips, back, abs, and upper body working together so that one body part doesn't strain and become injured. Since all movement comes from your center, we want to focus on strengthening there first.

CAUTION: People diagnosed with spinal stenosis—a narrowing of the vertebral space—should avoid extension exercises in general, but may be able to do them if properly supported. Seek advice from your doctor or physical therapist about precautions with exercise if you have this or any other degenerative condition of the spine.

Opposite Arm and Leg Extension (A) Quadruped

INSTRUCTIONS: Begin in table position on hands and knees with your wrists lined up under your shoulders and knees lined up directly under the hips. Find neutral position (rock your spine slightly between extension and flexion until you feel your abs fire and your back is flat. Imagine you have a glass of water on your back and you don't want it to spill). Now, extend one leg out behind you as if reaching to close a door with the heel of your foot. Your leg should be level with your shoulders. If you are struggling with your balance, just work on keeping neutral while you alternate leg extensions on each side. Once you can keep your neutral spine position here, you can add extension of the opposite arm.

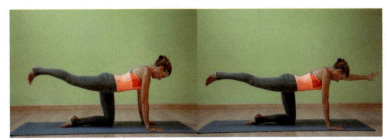

Fig. 30 Leg Extension   Fig. 30b Opposite Arm and Leg Extension

Hold for two to three breaths and work up to ten to twenty reps on each side.

NOTE: Be mindful of maintaining a neutral spine with these exercises. If you're wobbly or straining to hold the position, back down to an easier level until you master the move. It won't help you if you're doing it incorrectly.

Opposite Arm and Leg Extension (B) Prone

INSTRUCTIONS: For this one, you'll lie on your stomach with arms extended overhead. Tighten your abs and glutes, find neutral, and then lift one leg and the opposite arm. If this is too difficult and you feel as if you're straining, lift only one leg at a time. Then lift one arm at a time. Progress to opposite arm and leg extension when you can maintain neutral position while lifting each extremity individually. Hold for two to three breaths and repeat. Work up to ten to twenty reps on each side.

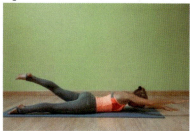

Fig. 55 Prone Opposite Arm and Leg Extension

ADVANCED: Once you've mastered the move, either on your hands and knees or on your belly, you can add a small hand weight (1-3 pounds) for added resistance. Don't compromise your form.

NOTE: Be careful to keep your head in a neutral position (chin tucked down, eyes on the mat) to avoid straining the neck. For people with lower back issues, try a folded towel or place a small pillow under the hips and lower belly. This exercise can also be done over a physio-ball if extension aggravates your lower back or you're uncomfortable lying on your stomach. The physio-ball is an excellent way to add an element of instability to your exercise routine, but it also requires more balance, so proceed with caution and seek advice from a trainer or physical therapist for instructions on proper use.

Crunches and Ab Work (Should I or shouldn't I?)

I have no objection to properly executed crunches and sit-up type exercises. There are real benefits to strengthening the abdominals in this way and tons of options. However, because we are dealing with bodies that sit so much, our abdominals and hip flexors are already prone to being in a shortened position, our shoulders are already rounded, and our neck muscles are often too weak to tolerate this additional abuse, causing us to strain and making it difficult to do the exercise correctly. So, for this text, we'll skip the military favorites, such as sit-ups, crunches, and leg lifts.

Go ahead; jump up and down in gratitude that I won't be assigning sit-ups and crunches as part of your regimen. But don't get too excited. We have an excellent alternative—known as *plank* work. Can you say **#ILovePlanks?** Don't panic. Planks are the one stop shop for anyone seeking to improve overall strength and stability, and there are such a wide variety of options for making them easier or harder, you'll never get bored. Here's the basic progression I recommend.

Quarter Plank

INSTRUCTIONS: Lie on your stomach on a firm surface (use a yoga mat for comfort). Prop onto your forearms so your elbows line up directly under your shoulders. Lengthen your upper arm bones to engage your serratus anterior (the muscles wrapping around your rib cage) and create space between your shoulder blades. This immediately sets you up for a firm base of support and works on the scapular stabilizers, which we will be talking about soon. Curl your toes under, tighten your abs and glutes by drawing your belly button into your spine and tucking your tailbone slightly downward, and lift just your belly and hips off the mat. You'll be on your knees in a flat back position. Hold for two to three breaths and lower slowly. Repeat. Work up to doing ten to twenty reps before moving on to half plank.

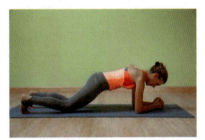

Fig. 56a Quarter Plank

NOTE: To increase the difficulty, alternately lift one knee off the floor and press out through the heel as shown below. Your focus should be on maintaining that flat back, plank position, so if your hips wobble when you lift one knee, you aren't quite ready for the progression to half plank.

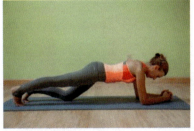

Fig. 56b Quarter Plank with Alternating Knee Lift

Half Plank

INSTRUCTIONS: Assume the same prone position as with quarter plank, resting on your forearms. Lengthen out the upper arm bones and engage the scapular stabilizers as before. Curl your toes under, draw the belly button in, tuck the tailbone down, and lift the belly and hips off the mat. This time, however, you'll also lift the knees so that your full weight will be on forearms and toes (balls of the feet). Hold for two to three breaths. Slowly lower to the floor, rest for a breath and repeat. Work up to ten to twenty reps before moving on to full plank. If you can only do a few, that's fine. Return to quarter plank as needed until you're stronger.

NOTE: To kick this up a notch, you can alternately touch one knee at a time to the mat, which will force you to engage your oblique abdominal muscles. Although this appears to be similar to the above noted progression, it requires an eccentric contraction (meaning the muscle has to stay contracted even as it elongates, aka. a negative contraction or deceleration movement). Trust me, it's harder, and very effective.

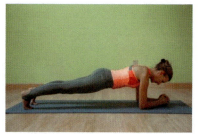

Fig. 57 Half Plank

Full Plank

INSTRUCTIONS: Begin on hands and knees in table position. Make those arm bones long again, but don't lock your elbows. Stretch one leg at a time out behind you, curl your toes under, and rise up onto hands and feet so that your body is in a straight line from head to heels. **Congratulations! You are in plank position.** Don't panic if you're a bit shaky or can't hold this position for long. Modify by coming onto your knees, but keep your back flat and hips in front of knees. The most important thing to remember is proper technique. Don't let the hips drop or stick up in the air. (It's helpful to do this in front of a mirror). Focus on the breath and build up slowly. Come down onto your knees and rock back into child's pose to rest between reps as needed.

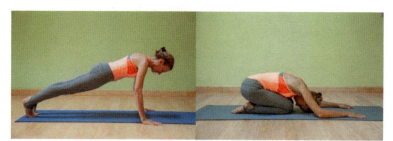

Fig. 35 Full Plank   Fig. 33a Rest in Child's Pose

ADVANCED: Once you master quarter plank, half plank, and full plank, and are able to do each with good form, you're ready for the fun stuff. Here are a few variations of plank that work on deeper stabilizing muscles as well as the larger muscle groups of the upper body and torso.

Side Plank

INSTRUCTIONS: From a full plank position, shift your weight onto one hand, making sure that your wrist is lined up directly under your shoulder. Rotate your body to one side, and raise your top arm toward the ceiling, turning your feet so that the top foot is in front of the bottom foot and you are weight bearing through the inner edge of the top foot and the outer edge of the bottom foot. Keep your abdominals tuned in and don't allow the hips to drop. If this is too difficult, place your bottom knee down on the mat for support.

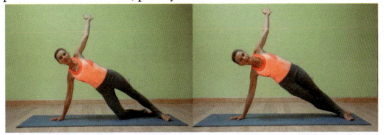

Fig. 58a Modified Side Plank   Fig. 58b Full Side Plank

MORE ADVANCED

Side Plank Crunches (Attempt side plank crunches only if you're able to hold a solid side plank with good form for thirty seconds.)

INSTRUCTIONS: You didn't think you'd get away without ANY crunches, did you? Repeat the steps for side plank as above. Place your free hand behind your head and draw your elbow across your body toward your opposite elbow, tightening your oblique abdominal muscles as you "crunch" into the movement. Return to top position and repeat, working up to ten to twenty reps on each side.

MODIFICATION: If this feels like a bit too much, feel free to modify by bending your lower leg and resting your knee onto the mat as noted in the above side plank modification illustration.

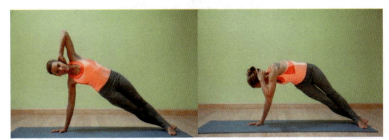

Fig. 59a and 59b Side Plank Crunch (Elbow toward elbow)

At this point you might be saying, but PJ…are you nuts? Well, a little. But if you've made it this far with the exercises, you're probably beginning to notice some changes in your body. Are you sitting up a little taller? Feeling a bit stronger? Are your pants fitting differently? Kudos! Stick with it. There's lots more to come and you're on your way to a healthier, happier you.

Let's move on to a few upper body strengthening exercises to help tone up those arms.

Upper Extremity Strengthening/Scapular Stabilization

WHY IT'S IMPORTANT: I mentioned earlier that I use the word "core" a bit differently than the average trainer. I see the entire trunk as your core rather than just the abdominals and lower back. After all, those upper back muscles are primarily responsible for giving you good posture and shouldn't be excluded, right? The latissimus dorsi, the largest of the back muscles (often referred to as your lats) connects from the underside of the upper arm all the way down into the lower back, and is one of the primary stabilizers of the spine during upper extremity activities.

In addition to the large upper back muscles such as the lats, traps, and rhomboids, there are scapular stabilizing muscles that work constantly when you're sitting. These muscles include your rotator cuff muscles, anterior serratus (those fan like muscles that wrap around your rib cage), levator scapulae, and pectoralis minor (not shown).

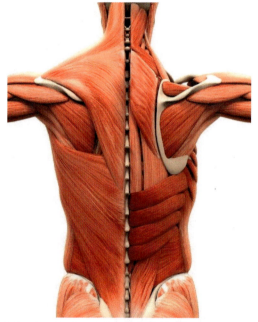

Fig. 60 Back of the body muscles involved in stabilizing the scapula

Weakness of these muscle groups contributes to the rounded shoulder/forward head posture that gets us into trouble. It can lead to impingement syndrome of the shoulder, rotator cuff tendinitis, carpal tunnel syndrome, upper extremity radiculopathy (numbness/tingling usually caused by nerve root or blood vessel entrapment), and a biomechanical reduction in upper extremity ROM and function.

In other words, weak scapular stabilizers make you slouch and can lead to pain, fatigue, and further loss of mobility.

Shoulder and Upper Back Exercises

Scapular Squeezes

INSTRUCTIONS: This exercise may be done sitting or standing. With palms up, thumbs pointing out, and elbows in at your side, slowly rotate your hands outward by externally rotating the shoulders, and squeeze your shoulder blades together. Return to neutral. Repeat ten times. **Doing this exercise several times per day will do wonders for counteracting the rounded shoulders of the desk dweller and strengthening the rotator cuff, thereby reducing risk of impingement syndrome in the shoulder.**

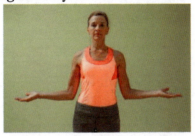

Fig. 61 Scapular Retraction

Bank Robber stretch

INSTRUCTIONS: Lean your back up against a blank wall with your heels a few inches away. Find your neutral spine position and keep your hips and upper back connected to the wall. Maintain the natural curve of your spine. Raise your arms out to the sides to just below a 90 degree angle with the elbows bent and back of the arms connected to the wall. Externally rotate your shoulders and try to reach the backs of your hands to the wall behind you. Don't worry if your hands don't touch at first. The tightness in your shoulders is preventing this, but over time, the muscles will stretch to allow full external rotation at the shoulders.

Keeping your elbows and the back of the arms connected to the wall as best you can, slowly raise and lower your hands in a "stick-em-up" motion. Repeat five to ten times. This is one of those exercises you can do in the shower, or even on a bed if you want to eliminate gravity and make it easier.

This is my go-to posture corrector!

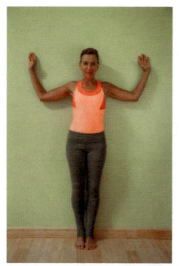

Fig. 62 Bank Robber Stretch
(Raise arms slowly up and down while keeping arms connected to wall)

Thera-band Exercises

Strengthening your rotator cuff and postural muscles of the upper back is essential for combatting the effects of prolonged sitting. If you don't take significant countermeasures, the long term toll will become evident in painful conditions that are difficult to reverse.

The following exercises can be done without resistance, but I recommend getting a light or medium Thera-tubing or resistive band. You can pick these up at your local sporting goods store or physical therapy office. Start with the lightest resistance and work up to stronger bands as tolerated.

Pull Downs

INSTRUCTIONS: Wrap your Thera-band securely around a solid object at about hip height. A stair railing works well or you can wrap it around the back of a doorknob and close the door tightly. You'll have both ends of the band to hold in each hand. Stand with your feet hip width apart, knees slightly bent. Engage your abdominals to find neutral position, and squeeze your shoulder blades back and down before pulling the Thera-band down to your hips. You don't need to pull past the seam of your pants. The idea is to engage the lats and scapular stabilizers, not to stress the posterior deltoid or engage the upper traps. Repeat two to three sets of ten to fifteen reps. (Start with ten reps and build up as tolerated.)

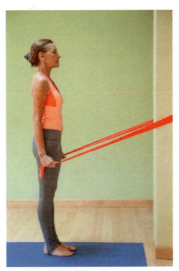

Fig. 63a Pull Down

Pull Back

INSTRUCTIONS: Secure the Thera-band as above and take each end in hand. Knees are slightly bent and neutral spine is engaged. This time, however, bend the elbows and draw the Thera-band straight back toward your ribs as if elbowing the guy behind you or pulling the reins on a horse. (Step back or wrap the band around your hands a few times to add resistance.) Squeeze the shoulder blades together and then release slowly.

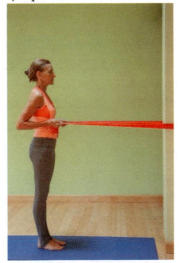

Fig. 63b Pull Back

External Rotation

INSTRUCTIONS: To work the external rotators, we'll do an exercise similar to the scapular retraction we did earlier, but now you're adding the resistance of a light Thera-band. With palms up, thumbs pointing outward, and elbows in at your sides, wrap the Thera-band around each hand and hold it in front of you. Squeeze the shoulder blades back and down and bring the hands apart, engaging the resistance of the Thera-band as you bring the hands just beyond a neutral position. Don't strain or struggle to bring the hands out wide. If you feel a pinching in the shoulders or find yourself arching your back and losing the neutral position, reduce your ROM. Build up slowly on repetitions with this one and listen to your body. You'll be amazed at how weak these muscles are and how quickly they fatigue. Start with five to ten reps and build up to two to three sets of ten.

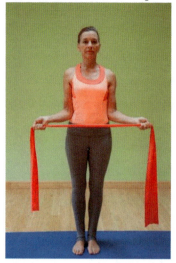

Fig. 64 External Rotation

Push Ups

WHY IT'S IMPORTANT: Doing push-ups might seem counterintuitive since I've spent this book lamenting about tight pecs and overworked neck and back muscles. But here's the thing;

Tight muscles are weak muscles.

When muscles are in a shortened position for long periods of time, they not only become tight, but they weaken because of their limited range of motion. Pushups work the muscles through their full range and require stabilizing muscles to fire throughout the body. When done properly, they are fantastic for sculpting, strengthening, and improving the stabilization capabilities of your neck, back, and shoulder muscles.

But PJ, you say, I've never done a push up in my life. They're just too hard. I say, poppycock! If you can master a full plank, you can progress to push-ups. Even if you haven't managed a full plank yet, you can begin with wall push-ups. The only caveat is that you need enough core stability and upper body strength to maintain good form. Here's my suggestion for a progression that will—before you know it—have you doing full military push-ups and feeling stronger than you've felt in years.

INSTRUCTIONS:

Wall push-ups—Place your hands on a firm wall or flat, empty surface (the side of the refrigerator or a door works if you can't find a blank wall.) Step up to the wall so that your toes are touching it and take two steps back, heel-to-toe so you're measuring two of your own foot lengths away from the wall. Next, widen your stance with feet hip width apart. With arms extended out straight, palms connected to the wall, I want you to feel as though you are doing a plank on the floor. Your abdominals are engaged, your spine is in the neutral position, and your head is in good alignment with the rest of your spine. Widen your hands to beyond shoulder width apart. You might need to make adjustments after the first one or two reps to get the hands just right. Bend your elbows and slowly lower yourself toward the wall (taking a breath in as you focus on maintaining a perfect plank position). Now exhale as you press your arms straight—without locking your elbows. Lower and lift ten to fifteen times and slowly build up to thirty reps (either three sets of ten or two sets of fifteen repetitions) before progressing to the next level.

NOTE: When you're in the full push-up position with arms bent and chest lowered toward the floor, your elbows should be over your wrists. Adjust your hand position as needed for proper alignment. Also, tuck your chin slightly in order to keep your cervical spine straight. No cricked necks! Push-ups are one of those exercises you could do every day, but since the shoulders and chest muscles of desk dwellers are tight anyway, I recommend doing push-ups every other day or about three times per week. Don't be concerned about making these muscles tighter. As stated above, tight muscles are weak muscles and we want our chest and shoulder muscles to be strong. As long as you are doing your stretches and upper back strengtheners as well, you'll keep things in balance.

If wall push-ups seem difficult or you're cursing me out after ten reps, cut it back to five and add a few repetitions each week until you can do them in sets of ten, giving yourself ten to fifteen second rests between sets as needed.

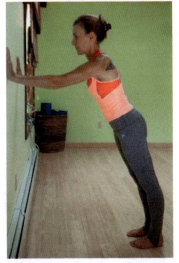

Fig. 65a Wall Push-up

Incline Push-ups—Repeat the steps above, but perform the push-ups at an angle. Countertop height is a good progression. Once you can do your thirty reps there, move on to a deeper angle until you can progress to a mat on the floor.

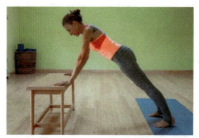

Fig. 65b Incline Push-ups

Modified push-ups—Begin on hands and knees in table position. Walk your hands forward of your shoulders and place them wider than shoulder width apart as above. Shift your weight forward, keeping a neutral spine by engaging your abdominals and maintaining a flat back or "plank" as you assume the push-up position. You can have your toes curled under or feet off the mat entirely, but you'll be weight bearing on your knees and hands. Lower slowly and then press back up, inhaling on the way down and exhaling as you rise. Avoid locking the elbows and be sure to keep your head in good alignment with the rest of your spine. Repeat in sets as above. If you can only do a few at first, that's okay. Build up slowly, adding a few reps a week until you can do ten in a row. Rest for ten to fifteen seconds between sets.

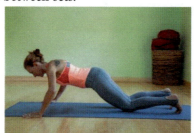

Fig. 66 Modified Push-up

Full (Military) Push-ups—Begin in table position with arms spread greater than shoulder width apart as above. Walk the hands forward, curl the toes under and press up into full plank. Widen your hand position to wider than shoulder width so the elbows line up over the wrists when you are in the "down" position of your push-up. Lower and raise your body, following the breath in as you lower and exhaling as you rise. If you're unable to maintain a solid plank position throughout the movement, go back to the modified version until you can. Quality verses quantity, right? Work up to two to three sets of ten to fifteen repetitions.

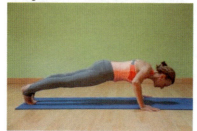

Fig. 67b Full Military Push-up

Neck Strengtheners

Isometrics—Isometrics might seem insignificant, but I assure you, they are effective when performed consistently, and should be a staple exercise in your battle to restore muscle balance to your cervical spine if you're having neck trouble. Isometrics are easily incorporated into your day and can be done anywhere, including while you're sitting at your desk or in your car…or even sitting on the potty—wherever you find yourself momentarily unoccupied. Get into the habit of doing them two to three times throughout the day. Perhaps when you take those water breaks or while you're sitting at a traffic light.

INSTRUCTIONS: Assume good posture with shoulders back and down and spine in a neutral position. Place two fingers on the left side of your forehead on the bony surface just anterior to your temple (**NOT on the soft part of the temple**). Gently press your forehead into your fingers and fingers into your forehead, meeting the resistance without letting your head turn to the left. This force without movement causes an **isometric contraction** of the cervical stabilizing muscles. Just a pound or two of pressure is needed to strengthen these muscles. If you're not sure of what one or two pounds of pressure is, press with two fingers on a bathroom scale or one of the hanging scales in the produce department of your grocery story. **NOTE: It doesn't require much effort, so if you are straining, trembling, losing your neutral position, or otherwise feeling discomfort, you're working too hard.** We don't want the larger muscles to be over firing. Instead, we want the smaller, weaker stabilizing muscles to do the work. This exercise is about retraining your cervical stabilizers to do the job of holding your head in the correct position.

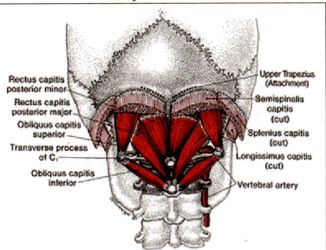

Fig. 68 Suboccipital Cervical Muscles

Hold for five seconds and repeat on the other side. Alternate giving resistance to the right, then the left, and repeat five times on each side, ensuring that you're maintaining a neutral position in both the neck and low back. It does no good to strengthen the muscles if you are slouching in the process.

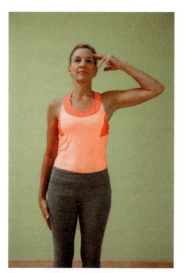

Fig. 69a Isometric Cervical Rotation

Add resisted forward flexion, extension, and side bending to the right and left. Repeat five times each, holding the isometric contraction for five seconds.

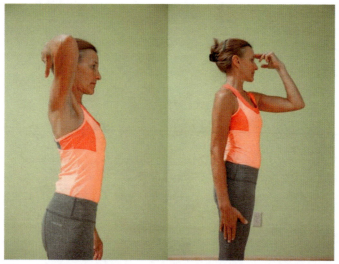

Fig. 69b Extension   **Fig. 69c Forward Flexion**

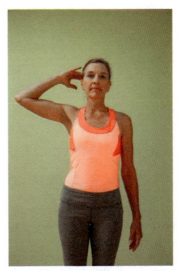

Fig 69d Resisted Lateral Flexion (Side Bending)

Chin Tucks

INSTRUCTIONS: I call this one the "chicken pecking" exercise. Have you ever watched chickens bob their heads forward and back as they strut around? It almost looks like their head is sliding forward and back on an even plane.

Assume your neutral position whether in sitting or standing. Tuck your chin in and slightly down as if someone has a string attached to the center of the back of your head and is drawing it backward. Next, glide your head forward on a horizontal plane as if you are reaching your nose forward. Be sure to keep the shoulders still and only move the head in a comfortable range of motion.

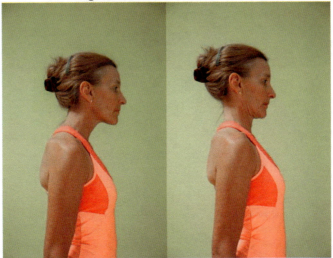

Fig. 70a and 70b Cervical Protraction and Retraction (Proper Chin Tuck)

Repeat five to ten times. This is another exercise that you could do two to three times daily and it would only improve your posture. The trick is in remembering to do these. I try to incorporate them into my sitting time at the computer or sometimes in the car. I can only imagine what other drivers think of me. Frankly, I don't care how I look. What matters is how I feel, and these exercises help me to continue living my life and being productive.

Restorative Poses

After exercise or at the end of a long day, I recommend assuming a restorative pose to allow muscles to relax, heart rate and blood pressure to come down, and for the mind and body to rest together in a contemplative state. The following are just a few such poses that can assist in reversing the negative effects of daily stress. If you suffer from edema in the lower extremities (swollen feet and ankles), the legs up the wall pose is especially helpful. Relaxing in these postures for a few minutes each will offer an energy balancing and restorative moment of relaxation any time you need it.

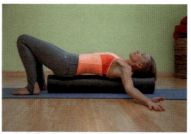

Fig. 71 Chest Stretch on Foam Roller

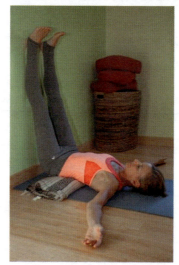

Fig. 72 Legs Up the Wall Pose

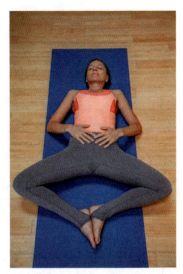

Fig. 73 Feet together, knees apart, hands on belly

Lessons in ADLs (activities of daily living)

We haven't worked specifically on leg strengthening yet, but I've included some functional training in this section that should help in that department. Lower extremity strengthening is beneficial for many reasons, not the least of which is that it's a requirement for actually getting up out of a chair or climbing stairs. Cultivating strong limbs and developing an understanding of how to maintain neutral position of your spine while performing ADLs will go miles for helping prevent injury and reduce the wear and tear on the joints of your spine. How many times have you, or someone you know, hurt themselves bending over to pick up something as insignificant as a set of dropped car keys. It wasn't only the odd bend and twist combo they did when they reached down, but it was the hundred other things they did "incorrectly" that day that set them up for the injury. Think about how many times a day we bend forward without considering our body mechanics. And don't forget about the four hundred pounds of pressure repeatedly placed on our low back each time we lean the upper body out beyond our toes without bending our knees. Suffice it to say, we need strong legs and a strong core, and we need to know how to use them properly to protect our spine.

Proper Squats

WHY IT'S IMPORTANT: Learning to squat and lunge properly and applying them to ADLs such as lifting laundry baskets, emptying the trash, and carrying groceries (or children), will save your back and neck much grief and aggravation. Practicing these moves on a regular basis will also lead to obtaining that lean body we'd all like to have. Incorporate sets of chair squats and lunges into your ten minute mini workouts throughout the day.

> **Lean muscle mass is a keystone to a healthy metabolism and maximizes your body's fat burning potential.**

NOTE: If you have knee or hip issues, I recommend modifying squats and lunges by reducing the range of motion (don't squat or lunge as deeply), and always remember to keep the knee in line with the ankle. NEVER allow the knee to go out past the toes. If you're still having pain after modifying the exercise, seek guidance from a physical therapist or personal trainer for tips on technique, or skip it all together.

When executed correctly with modifications, you should be able to do some version of this exercise. It may also be that you need to work on more basic strengthening activities such as straight leg raises or minimal wall squats before progressing to deeper squats and lunges. Another option is to do them in a pool where the buoyancy allows for greater pain-free range of motion and limited weight-bearing.

INSTRUCTIONS: Stand in front of a stationary chair or countertop (nothing with wheels), with your feet wider than shoulder width apart and your toes slightly turned out. Bend at your knees and hinge at your hips as if you are reaching your bottom out behind you to sit in the chair. It may feel as if your weight is through your heels and that you might tip backwards, but if you reach with your arms out in front of you, your weight should be counterbalanced.

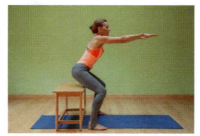

Fig. 75 Proper Squatting Technique

Keep your head up with eyes facing front, shoulders down and back and chest lifted. **Your knees should not come forward of your toes.** Your goal is to be able to touch your bottom to the edge of the seat and come back up. Add a glute squeeze at the top for extra toning. Repeat in sets of five to ten reps, adding a set every few days until you are able to do thirty reps. It may take time to build up to this and as a I mentioned above, quality trumps quantity, so if you're getting fatigued and sloppy with the execution, STOP! Mindfulness is your best friend here. Pay attention and move through the exercise slowly. Don't worry about the numbers. Do it correctly and build up as tolerated.

Lunges

INSTRUCTIONS: With your hands on your hips, take a step forward with your left foot. Give yourself a wide base of support. In other words, if your feet are in a straight line one in front of the other, balance is going to be difficult, so be sure to have your feet set apart. The distance between your feet from front to back is also an individual consideration. You want to be sure that when you sink into your lunge your front knee is over your ankle and not over your toes. This exercise can be done next to a countertop so you can hold on to something stationary if balance is a problem.

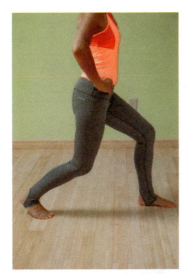

Fig. 76 Proper Lunge Position

Once your feet are set and your balance is steady, lower the back knee toward the floor. You'll want to keep your shoulders over your hips and back straight. The weight will be in the heel of the front foot and on the ball of the back foot. Step the feet together and repeat on the other side. Take it slow, but try to find a pace and rhythm that allows you to flow through the movement. You'll actually find it easier than going super slow. It helps to count out the steps.

1. Step forward
2. Bend the back knee and lower it toward the floor
3. Come back up
4. Bring the feet together

Practical application of these movements for ADLs

Squats and lunges are versatile tools for any time you find yourself lifting a laundry basket, a box of books, or a small child. If you're leaning forward and feeling stress on your neck or back, check in with your new "biomechanics meter" and see if squatting or lunging will be more efficient for your task than bending at the waist. Think of how it felt to do the Dead Bug exercise where you had to maintain neutral position while moving your arms and legs simultaneously. Employ those same principles of maintaining neutral position while you're performing overhead lifting activities or are reaching away from your center for any reason.

Avoid bending and twisting motions and know your weight limit for lifting. Think like MacGyver when it comes to moving heavy items. How can you use things around your household to make the job easier? Step stools, rolling carts, dollies, and pulley systems can be useful additions to any home projects requiring might, but don't let your pride get you into trouble. Ask for help if you need it.

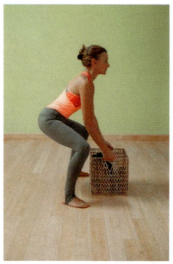

Fig. 4 Proper Lifting Position

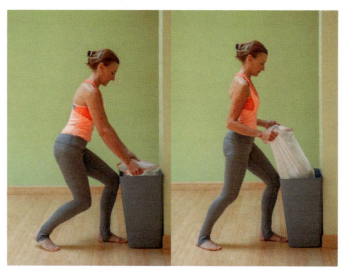

Fig. 77a and 77b
Use your lunge position for things like removing a trash bag from the bucket, gardening, or vacuuming.

Now that you're stronger and more flexible, put those new muscles to good use and start living your life. Get outside, become active, learn to manage your time, and remember what's important. Do your best to incorporate exercise into every part of your life. Recognize that your best will be different from day to day. Some days you'll feel as if you're losing the battle, but hang in there. Once armed with all the right tools and endless positive choices, you'll find it easier to get back up and move forward toward your goals again. The foundation to living a full life is to maintain a healthy body. Without that, everything becomes harder. Your daily activities overwhelm and exhaust you, relationships suffer, your job suffers, and worst of all…you suffer. Information is power. You've taken the first step by reading this book. In the next section we'll talk about more ways you can improve the quality of your life with simple self-care techniques.

CHAPTER 12

TREATMENT AND SELF CARE

There are so many creative and wonderful ways you can care for your own neck and back problems. Stretching and strengthening exercises and healthy nutrition are only the beginning. In this section I'll be discussing several treatment approaches, which are easily implemented and can be done most anywhere. We'll start with my favorite topic...

MASSAGE

Good books on self-massage abound, but for the purposes of this text, I'll focus on what I find to be the most effective techniques and self-care tools in my arsenal. If you've ever had a sore muscle, you know the instinct is to rub it, knead it like a lump of clay, or dig into it as if you're trying to surgically remove the knots with your fingers and thumbs. Although this shotgun approach can have some benefit and offer temporary relief, it usually doesn't get to the underlying problem, and your hands and fingers probably give out before the knots do. Moreover, if you don't know what you're looking for, you can actually do more harm than good.

MASSAGE BASICS

I tell my clients that massage shouldn't "hurt," and if it does, to tell me. More specifically, I tell them on a scale of 1-10, ten being *"don't ever do that to me again,"* and one being, *"you're hardly touching me,"* a "5-6" is as much as you need to tolerate to have it be effective. If the discomfort is making you hold your breath or tighten up, it's too much. I also check in frequently to be sure they aren't just toughing it out. Massage should be relaxing and rejuvenating. If you drink plenty of water after your massage and don't do something crazy like bungee jumping or vacuuming the whole house afterward, you shouldn't feel like a train hit you the next day. Keep this in mind when you work on yourself. More is not better. With practice, you'll discover *therapeutic depth* and learn to work with that in mind.

NOTE: Manipulation of soft tissue releases toxins and water helps flush those toxins out, so drink at least eight 8-ounce glasses the day of and the day after your massage. Even if you're working on yourself, the trick is to stay hydrated (remember; wine, coffee, and soda do not count).

Massage can be done anytime and anywhere. I find myself working on my neck in the car, at conferences, in movie theatres...pretty much whenever it's bugging me, I'm treating it in some way. I use the pads of my fingers and massage in circular motions along the thick para-spinal muscles on either side of my neck, working up and down the length of the muscle from the base of my skull down to my upper traps on both sides. Rubbing and pressing on the attachments at the base of the skull can have an amazing affect. The layers of muscle and fascia that weave into the scalp are a complex web of connective tissue that can bind down against the flat bones of the cranium and cause a multitude of symptoms.

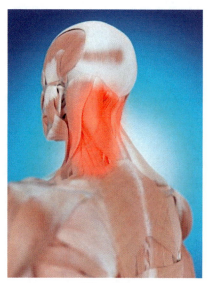

Fig. 78

Lack of hydration and lubrication, chronic muscle tension, and biomechanical influences wreak havoc on the head and neck. Regular massage to these areas can offer great relief from chronic headaches and even tension related migraines. Think about how good it feels when the hairdresser washes your hair and massages your scalp. Recreate that warm fuzzy sensation yourself by doing the following:

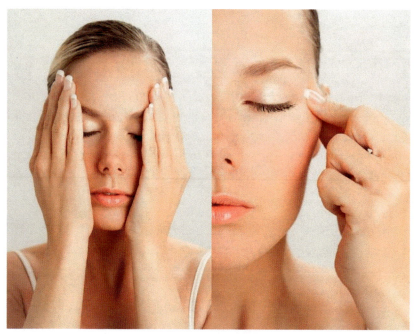

Fig. 79a and 79b

Rub your palms together to create heat in your hands. Take a few deep breaths and feel the energy intensify. Then gently rest your warm palms over your eyes. Hold here for a breath or two and feel the tension ease. With the pads of your fingertips, massage in small, circular motions around the eyes and along the eyebrows, out toward the temple. Massage the temples with gentle circles. Moving around to the side of your head, focus on the temporalis muscle above the ears. If you notice this area is particularly tight and tender, spend a few minutes here, gently working on the tender spots or holding them until you feel the tension ease.

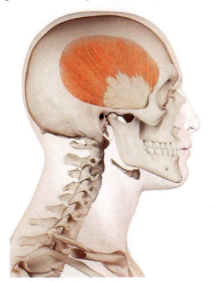

Fig. 80 Temporalis Muscle

Continue on to the forehead, massaging the frontalis muscle above the brows.

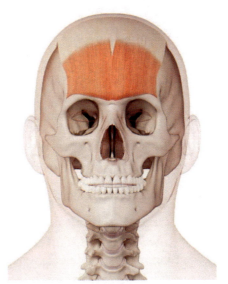

Fig. 81 Frontalis Muscle

Massage and gently press and hold the sinus points along the bridge of the nose and under the eyes.

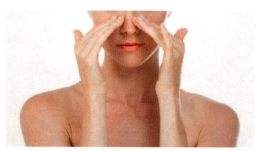

Fig. 82 Sinus Points

Pay special attention to the large masseter muscle that clenches the jaw.

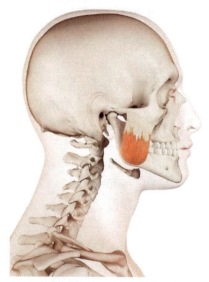

Fig. 83 Masseter Muscle

The masseter is our primary "chewing muscle," but we also contract this muscle instinctively when we're stressed and often unconsciously when we sleep. All that daily tension has to go somewhere, right? Teeth grinding is one clue that you are clenching. Chronic headaches are another sign. You can address this with your dentist, wear a night guard, and/or do some massage and gentle stretches for your jaw before bed. I also highly recommend finding a productive outlet for your stress.

NOTE: Teeth clenching can be a stress response, but it can also be about pent up, unexpressed emotion—especially anger. Suppressed anger has powerful negative effects on the body. Learning to deal with this emotion in a constructive manner and expressing it in some positive way is essential to health and well-being. Left to grow unchecked, negative emotions are like a ticking time bomb, waiting to destroy you from the inside out. High blood pressure, depression, migraines, ulcers, irritable bowel syndrome, and even cancer can result from stuffing toxic emotions. Exercise, psychotherapy, Cognitive Behavioral Therapy, and meditation are just a few ways to conquer the monster within. It takes courage to face our demons, express long-held emotions, and learn new coping skills, but the journey to peace and wellness is worth the effort.

The chronic muscle tension in your upper trap may be there courtesy of your wayward teen, pill of a boss, or nagging Aunt Josephine, as well as from your poor posture, so don't negate the effects of emotional "stressors" on the body. We'll talk more about stress management soon.

TRIGGER POINT RELEASE TECHNIQUE

On the physical level, those knots you seek to excise are known as trigger points. A trigger point—to keep it simple—is a group of irritated nerve endings in a muscle. I explain it to my clients like this:

The job of the blood supply is to carry oxygen-rich blood to all the cells in our body and to carry away toxins and waste products, allowing them to be filtered out through the liver, kidneys, lymphatic and excretory systems. When muscles stay tight for long periods of time, the blood flow is restricted and the toxins build up in the tissue and cause inflammation at the nerve endings, leading to pain. Proper hydration, healthy nutrition, consistent stretching, aerobic exercise, and massage are only a few tools we have to alleviate this problem. Since we're talking about massage techniques, let's discuss how we can find and release these trigger points with just the press of a finger, a thumb, or a "Back Buddy" aka, a Thera-cane.

INSTRUCTIONS: Not surprisingly, the most obvious trigger points may be found in your neck and shoulders, so we'll start there. Sit supported in a comfortable chair with feet flat and perhaps a lumbar pillow at your back. Rest your left hand over your right shoulder/neck area. Begin by gently squeezing your upper trapezius muscle using the heel of your hand and the flat of all your fingers, kneading up and down the muscle a few times to increase the circulation locally while also surveying the area to find the most tender spots. **NOTE: Support your right elbow by cradling it in the left hand so you can relax as much as possible (not shown).**

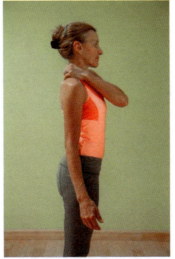

Fig. 84 Kneading Right Upper Trap

Press your index or middle finger (which I find is stronger and more sensitive) into the muscle, working across the length of the upper trap in a grid like fashion, moving the finger a half inch at a time along a line from the base of the neck to the tip of the shoulder. These "finger presses" alone can be helpful in alleviating muscle tension. Stop when you hit a tender spot. Press in a bit deeper until you feel a radiation of the pain to an area away from the actual spot. This radicular or remote pain reference is the hallmark of a trigger point. If you're pressing into the upper trap and feel an achy sensation move up into the back of the head, down into the shoulder blade, or shoot over the top of your head and land behind your eye, you're on the right track!

Hold the trigger point for 30-60 seconds. There is much debate about how long trigger points take to "dissolve" or dissipate, but I've found that holding until you feel a pulsation or release, is sufficient. If you held for the full recommended ninety seconds (as with Jones TP releases) you might be in for a long session. I find that trigger points tend to hang out in clusters and that moving the fingers in ever widening circles will land you on several more trigger points that need attention, each one offering more relief than the last. Work on an area for a few minutes and then move on. No digging. You're not trying to bruise yourself or injure the tissue.

Press-Hold 30-60 seconds-Breathe-Release

NOTE: As you press on the TP, it might help to slowly rotate the head side to side to create a pin-and-stretch effect, requiring less pressure and assisting the release. Listen to your body. The kind of pain you feel when releasing trigger points is one of those "good" pains. It's uncomfortable, but tolerable, and you should be able to maintain your breathing throughout the process.

Repeat this procedure along each upper trap. Move on to the upper back, toward another troubled area, the levator scapulae, rhomboids, and latissimus dorsi.

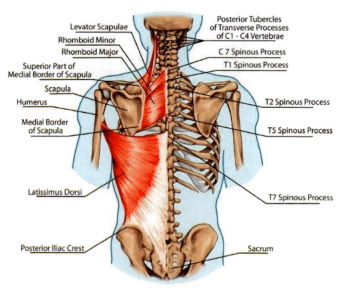

Fig. 85

Attending to these areas can become problematic as they aren't easily reached without tensing other muscles in the process. Short of leaning against the sharp edge of a door frame, lying on a tennis ball, or asking your partner to have a go at them, we need an effective trigger point eraser.

That's where my Back Buddy, the Thera-cane, comes in handy. You can pick up one of these nifty tools at the manufacturer's website or get it on Amazon for about $30. It's worth its weight in bonbons! **NOTE: I recommend the full S shaped tool rather than just the "hook" as I seem to be able to get better leverage and it has more options.** It comes with instructions on all the specific uses, but suffice it to say, it's like having an extension to your own fingers, or almost like having a personal massage therapist on staff…almost. You still have to become proficient with its use and practice good judgement about how much pressure to exert and where.

CAUTION: Stay off of bony prominences and areas where nerve bundles reside, such as the back of the knee, inner elbow, under the arm, inner thigh, and the carotid and trachea areas of the throat. If there's any question about where these are, consult an anatomy book or ask your massage therapist/PT to show you the danger zones to avoid.

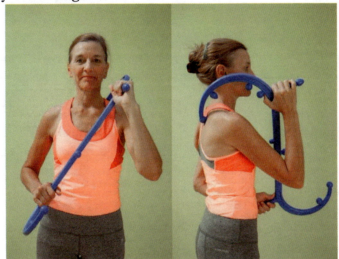

Fig. 86a and Fig. 8 Thera-cane Grip Front and Side View

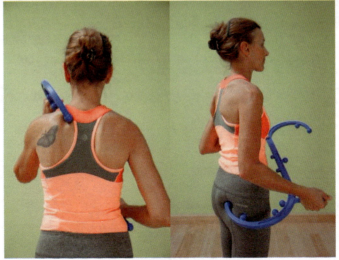

Fig. 86b and 86c Levator Scapulae and Piriformis Trigger Points

Again, be gentle with this tool. In the wrong hands, it can easily become a weapon. Releasing trigger points is—forgive the expression—a painstaking process. It takes patience, body awareness, and mindfulness. With practice, this tool can easily become the desk dweller's best friend. I keep mine next to the couch and use it a few times a week while catching up on my favorite shows. It tides me over between massage appointments and offers significant relief from those stubborn, hard to reach trigger points.

NOTE: Trigger points are tricky to eliminate completely since we can't avoid all the stresses on our body. Once TP's become chronic, management is our best plan of attack. It's also important to remember that the pain you feel is often connected to trigger points with remote locations, so to alleviate pain, we sometimes have to search for its origins. My "neck pain" for instance, is usually caused by trigger points around my scapula.

Other problem areas prone to trigger points are the back of the shoulder, lower back, hip and gluteal muscles, and even the bottoms of the feet.

NOTE: Massaging your feet once or twice a week can improve your over-all health tremendously since the Reflexology points in the soles of your feet correlate to all the organ systems of the body. Keeping your feet healthy and those energy channels open is essential for wellness. Consulting a reflexology chart can be helpful, or seek treatment from a Reflexology practitioner.

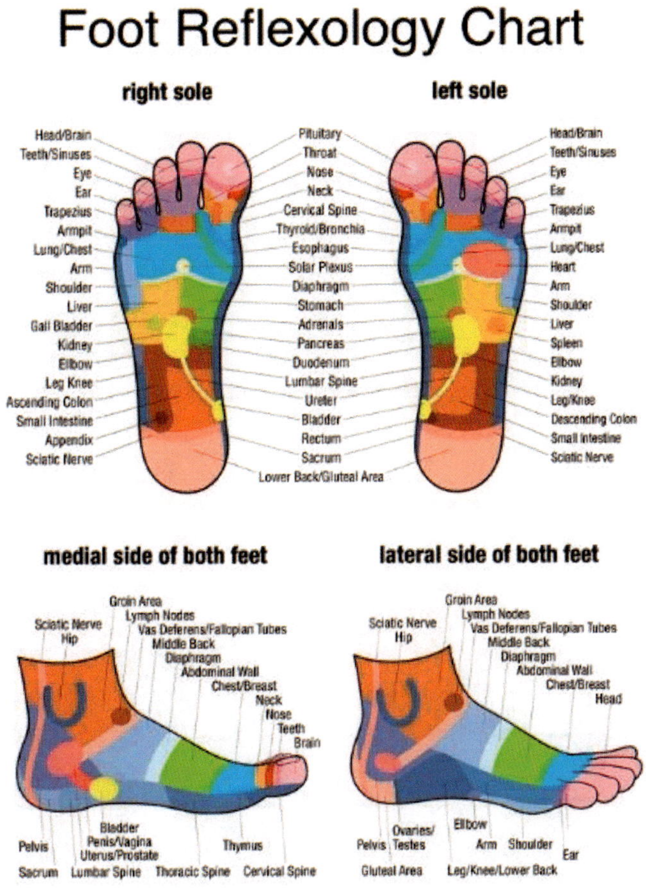

Foot Reflexology Chart

Fig. 87 Reflexology Chart

Your feet do so much for you, the least you can offer them is five or ten minutes of your attention a couple of times per week.

Help for creaky necks and "sticky" vertebrae

Before we leave the subject of manual therapy entirely, let me mention a few more techniques for neck care. If you already have neck pain, you've probably also noticed the creakiness in those joints when you try to turn your head after staring at the computer for an hour or more. It almost sounds like crinkling aluminum foil, doesn't it? I fondly refer to this as "Velcro Neck." Basically, when we're stationary for long periods of time, the synovial fluid that lubricates the joints becomes stagnant and "sticky." Usually a little movement—as with the neck exercises I've suggested—will reduce the "creaking" and you'll be able to resume normal function. But if you've been at this sedentary lifestyle thing for years, you're one of those people whose cervical spine doesn't stay in alignment well, or the biomechanics of the joints is compromised by muscle imbalances and arthritic changes, the range of motion deficits might be making their way to a more permanent state.

To avoid this, you can do a simple **mobilization** technique on yourself. People worry when they hear the word mobilization, connecting it immediately to chiropractic manipulation. But there are multiple grades of force used with mobilization techniques. Generally speaking, what a chiropractor or osteopath would typically use, would be considered high velocity manipulation. They bring the joint to its end range of motion and apply overpressure to make an adjustment. In physical therapy, joint mobilizations are used to increase range of motion of joints and normalize connective tissue that has scarred down or adhered, such as with frozen shoulder (adhesive capsulitis) or post-surgery. Here, they would use steady pressure, gentle oscillations and stretching to loosen the joint and get it moving. PTs also do spinal mobilizations, but this is not considered a manipulation as much as it is categorized as manual therapy since the force applied is a steady pressure designed to increase length of soft tissue structures and improve joint mobility rather than a forceful realignment of the joint.

Treatment might also include muscle energy techniques (also known as neuromuscular facilitation). Or manual traction to increase the space between vertebrae and reduce compression of discs and entrapment of nerve roots. Physical therapists are also often great resources for more subtle manipulations of the spine, using modalities such as craniosacral therapy to improve the flow of cerebrospinal fluid and myofascial release techniques to free up fascial restrictions. Much pain relief can be achieved with these therapies. Find a good manual therapist and it's like finding a trusted mechanic. You'll never take your car/body anywhere else.

Mulligan Mobs with Movement

The mobilization technique I'll share with you was developed by a physical therapist in Australia named Brian Mulligan. He teaches a whole series of techniques for restoring normal joint function, but this one is my go-to exercise for gentle cervical mobilizations I can do myself to "unstick" those cranky cervical vertebrae.

INSTRUCTIONS: Sitting up straight in neutral position, rest your right hand on the back of your neck, thumb pointing downward. Curl your fingers around the "fleshy part" of the left side of your neck, gently pressing your fingertips into the space just beyond your left cervical para-spinal muscles. I call this hand position a "monkey's paw" since the fingers are only bent at the distal two joints. The knuckle joints, aka MCP's (metacarpal phalangeal joints), are straight and aligned with the wrist.

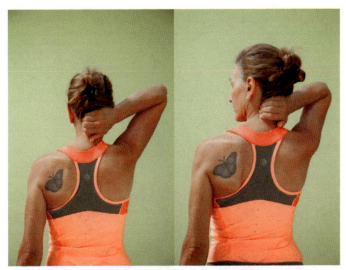

Fig. 88a and 88b Mulligan Mobilizations

Pulling gently in an upward motion with your fingers (about a 30 degree angle), rotate your head to the left. The hand is guiding the neck into the motion with a very slight overpressure. Return your head to center, move your fingers down a half inch and repeat. Progress down the spine like this until you reach the C7 vertebrae (the one that is usually most prominent at the base of the neck) and then work your way up again. Try to keep the movements smooth and fluid. Back and forth, back and forth, moving up and down the cervical spine 2-3x and then repeat on the opposite side. This gentle mobilization with movement "unlocks" the joints and assists them in their natural movement. You might even get a small click or pop as the joints adjust and begin to move more freely.

REFERENCE: For more of Mulligan's techniques to aid with headaches, vertigo, nausea and other vertebral artery signs, refer to his book, Manual Therapy, Nags, Snags, MWMS etc. by Brian R Mulligan.

MORE NECK HELPERS

Sub-occipital Release

We already talked about those tight muscle attachments at the base of your skull and how trigger points form in muscles and tendons. It just so happens that trigger points love to settle into these thick, fibrous attachments. An excellent way to release several at once, while also doing a cranial release is called **sub-occipital release**. This is typically done by a massage therapist or physical therapist by positioning their fingertips under the occiput and allowing gentle traction and the weight of your head to do the job of releasing the muscle tension at the attachments.

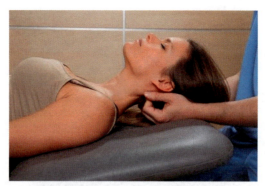

Fig. 89 Suboccipital Release

For at home do-it-yourselfers, there are devices called **"still point" inducers,** which can be purchased on line for about $20. Or you can MacGyver a perfectly suitable substitute by stuffing two tennis balls in a sock, tying off the end tightly, and lying with your head resting on the tennis balls **(position them so they're on either side of the spine at the base of the skull)** for about five minutes or until you feel the tension in your neck and head release. This is a great technique if you suffer from chronic headaches due to muscular tightness and stress.

Self-Muscle Energy Techniques (METs)

Another manual therapy technique I use on myself is considered a **self-muscle energy technique**. This one is a life saver. Maybe not my actual life, but perhaps my sanity. When my neck is out of alignment, I get headaches, whether from the stress of the muscle imbalance or the actual position of the vertebra placing pressure on nerves. They aren't migraines, and nothing truly debilitating, (probably because I treat myself immediately whenever possible), but annoying enough to make me want to take something along the lines of an over the counter NSAID or pain reliever.

Since I like to avoid meds that could have a negative effect on my stomach, kidneys, and liver, I like to reserve my use of pain relievers for real necessity. My headache is usually the first sign that something in my neck isn't quite aligned properly, so although a pain medication or anti-inflammatory might give me short term relief, it's not going to fix the problem.

Instead of popping pills, I sit up straight, assume the neutral position, and test my cervical rotation looking over one shoulder, then the other. If I've been at the computer for a while and "forgotten" to take a break, I can expect some creaking and crunching. Inevitably, it's painful and restricted in one direction or sometimes at the end range in both directions, and I wonder why I hadn't noticed this before. Clearly too much time had passed since I'd used this strange swiveling motion of my head. In fact, if I weren't a fanatic about stretching, I probably wouldn't have noticed the restriction until I tried to look over my shoulder when backing out of the driveway.

Don't ignore pain! It's telling you something, and if you don't pay attention and try to fix it, the pain will find a way to scream louder. Trust me on this. The principle of METs is simple, but the execution of the technique is a bit complex at first. If you want to skip the most "technical" part of this book,

now's your chance. For those of you suffering with painful limitations of your cervical spine, read on.

NOTE: Muscle energy techniques (METs) are a form of osteopathic manipulative diagnosis and treatment—in which the patient actively contracts their muscles from a precisely controlled position, in a specific direction, and against a counterforce applied at a specific intensity. METs are used to treat decreased range of motion, muscular hypertonicity, and pain. Learning muscle energy techniques is a complicated process and usually requires years of study and practice to master. There are many variables to consider and an understanding of anatomy, physiology, and biomechanics is usually necessary to become proficient with METs. On the other hand, the underlying principle is, as I said, simple, so here is your crash course in a self-muscle energy technique for increasing cervical range of motion and improving cervical alignment.

The following is a basic version of a contract-relax technique that I've found works for most people. The concept can be applied to any area of motion restriction as long as you have an understanding of what you are trying to accomplish (which muscles you want to lengthen to increase your ROM), and the movements involved in getting you there.

The good news is that if it doesn't work for you, it also won't likely make things worse, and even if you do this backward (an indirect, but equally effective technique), you'll probably get some positive results. If it doesn't reduce your pain or increase ROM, you may have a "locked" facet joint, or you need more than just a quick fix to get your cervical spine aligned properly and moving again.

CAUTION: If you're experiencing radiculopathy (pain, numbness, or tingling down the arm), the shotgun approach is **NOT** for you! This technique shouldn't be painful, so if you experience an increase in pain while doing it, stop and consult your doctor, physical therapist, or chiropractor for appropriate treatment.

HOW IT WORKS: For this example, let's say you're having pain and motion restriction when rotating your head to the right, meaning, you can't turn as far to the right as you can to the left, and movement in one direction or the other causes pain. This is not necessarily because the muscles are shorter or tighter on one side or the other (although they may be and often are), it's usually an indicator that there is a biomechanical dysfunction of the joints as well. **Using the contraction and subsequent relaxation of the muscles to affect joint mobility is the principle behind METs.**

We'll be employing a basic contract/relax technique (also known as reciprocal inhibition or post-isometric relaxation). The theory is twofold. Contraction of one muscle causes the opposing muscle to relax, allowing for greater flexibility of the primary muscle when you then try to stretch it. A secondary principle is that maximum contraction of a muscle is followed by maximum relaxation. This is important if the tight muscle is holding a bone in a misaligned position. By "taking up the slack" or moving toward a restricted range of motion, stopping at the edge of the barrier and contracting the opposing muscles, the bone is "pulled" back into alignment in incremental stages. In actuality, the bone is being "allowed" to return to its normal position. This is a very simplistic explanation of a complex reflex arc, but hopefully, you get the idea. Don't worry if your eyes are crossing. I'll break it down into simple steps.

Remember those isometrics we did in the exercise section? We're going to use them here. We're also going to refer to the six movements of the spine we discussed earlier when talking about range of motion: flexion, extension, right rotation, left rotation, right side bending and left side bending (aka; lateral flexion).

Since you aren't a professional, and you'll be making judgment calls about what is meant by **a precisely controlled position, in a specific direction, and against a counterforce applied at a specific intensity,** the term "precise" goes out the window—which is why I call this a "shotgun" approach.

Whether muscles are tight or weak, or some combination of the two, makes no difference here. You simply need to understand that a **"tight muscle will pull the joint into a dysfunctional position, and the weak muscle will allow it to happen."** Although I'm asking you to make assumptions about the positional diagnosis of a musculoskeletal dysfunction, **all you really need to know is in what motion are you restricted?**

I also expect you to use good judgment about how much counterforce to initiate to get the job done, so don't go crazy! Although I referred to "maximal" contraction above, it really takes minimal effort and force to achieve the desired result since we're working with relatively small muscles. A mere two pounds of pressure is all you need. Again, if you have no idea what two pounds feels like, find a scale and gently press two fingers onto the scale platform until the needle registers two pounds.

Don't be overzealous with the "more is better mentality." Think "baby fingers" or how hard you could press on a child's fingers without hurting them. (No testing this out on your children, please.)

INSTRUCTIONS: Ok, don't be scared. This is easy. Just follow the instructions and don't forget to breathe. We'll break it down into a four part process, so begin with small movements into each range of motion and progress to greater range with each repetition, working within your limitations. The idea is that you want to slowly take up the barrier presented by the restriction.

Here's how to do it:

In sitting, assume neutral position. Flex your head slightly forward (20% of your available motion), rotate your head slightly (20%) to the right as if looking at your armpit (towards the restricted side), and side bend slightly (20%) toward the right (as if bringing the right ear toward the right shoulder).

Place two fingers on the bony part of the left side of your forehead and gently resist against your fingers as if you want to turn your head to the left but your fingers won't let you move. This is an **isometric contraction.**

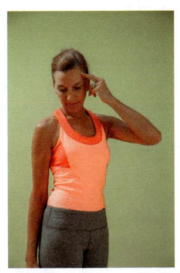

Fig. 90 Self-MET to Increase Right Rotation

Be gentle! Remember these are small muscles we're working with here. Hold for 6-10 seconds, then relax and move slightly deeper into each movement (flexion, rotation, and side bending to the right). **Each repetition, you'll add another approximation of about 10-20% of your available ROM in those three movements, *"listening"* to your body's limitations and letting them guide you. NO moving into pain.**

Give resistance to the left again with two fingers on the bony part of your forehead, hold for 6-10 seconds, and then repeat the process one more time, flexing, rotating, and side bending right, and then gently resisting to the left (for a total of three repetitions.)

Before returning to center, add one more component to the technique by placing your two fingers just above the left ear and resisting into left side bending as if bringing your left ear toward your left shoulder, but your fingers won't allow you to move. Hold for 6-10 seconds. Finish the technique by turning the head as far to the right as it will go comfortably, guiding it with the fingertips on the left side of the forehead, exerting a slight stretch at end range.

Return to center and retest your ROM. You should notice an increase in mobility and a decrease in pain. Repeat the sequence on the other side as needed if your motion is restricted or painful to that side as well. If it's still painful, try again, but don't force it. This technique can be done as often as needed to realign the cervical spine or increase cervical ROM. Recurrent restrictions in the same direction often happen with chronic neck pain so using muscle energy may become a staple in your efforts to keep your spine properly aligned.

Treating Your Back

Treating your own back can be a bit more challenging. Especially because we're limited by the difficulties inherent in accurate self-assessment and lack of familiarity of the anatomy and physiology of the musculoskeletal system. Even a degree in physics won't help you here. There are lots of moving parts, nerve bundles and layers upon layers of muscles.

When someone comes to see me complaining of back pain, I can look at their spine, assess their alignment and accompanying motion restrictions, and intuitively know the techniques I need to perform to correct any imbalances or mal-alignments. Years of practice and continuing education has given me the tools I need to assess and treat a multitude of musculoskeletal problems. If I see clients on a regular basis, I'll discover patterns that are problematic that have become chronic.

In other words, they "go out" of alignment the same way each time. Once I understand the pattern and what techniques to use to fix it, I can teach my clients simple self-MET's to correct it on their own. My clients have thanked me for this gift more times than I can count. Since you can't all come to my office, and there aren't enough pages in this book to teach you to do these techniques yourself, I'll try to give you a few tricks you can apply at home.

Releasing trigger points in the piriformis, glutes, and Quadratus lumborum (a lower back muscle responsible for laterally flexing and rotating the lumbar spine) can do wonders for reducing low back pain, since these muscles attach at the pelvis, sacrum, and lumbar vertebrae.

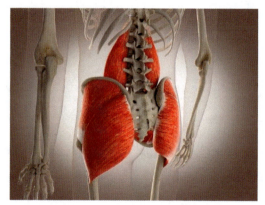

Fig. 91
Gluteus and Quadratus lumborum muscles
(Piriformis not shown, as it lies beneath the glutes)

You can use the Thera-cane, sit/roll on a tennis ball, or use a foam roller. Even knuckles and thumbs work as great tools for finding the trigger points that seem to collect in glutes, hips and low back. Working these out and stretching them is often enough to completely alleviate back pain.

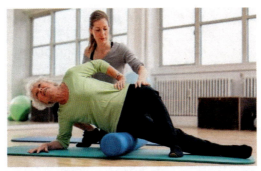

Fig. 92 Right ITB Release and Left Piriformis Stretch

NOTE: Please seek the advice of a physical therapist or personal trainer familiar with the many uses of a foam roller. It's an excellent tool for decreasing tightness of hard to stretch places like the Iliotibial Band (ITB, which runs along the outside of your leg from hip to knee), and deep hip musculature like the piriformis. As with any device, the foam roller requires proper use to be effective and professional instruction can reduce risk of injury.

Don't forget about the hip flexors in the front of the body as well. Since these thick and usually tight muscles attach into the lower back, they are a main source of lower back pain and contribute to malalignment issues. Working on trigger points in the anterior hip and abdomen can also offer significant relief from low back pain.

Piriformis Syndrome and Sciatica

The chronic pain in your butt that is not your Aunt Josephine is often caused by compression of the sciatic nerve, either from a bulging disc or due to a tight/inflamed piriformis muscle.

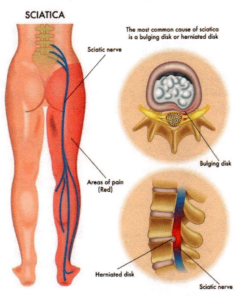

Fig. 93
Bulging Disc Causing Sciatica

If a bulging disc is the culprit, it's likely that sitting makes it worse and extension exercises, like press ups (cobra pose in yoga), relieve the symptoms. Bulging discs and sciatica can be treated with physical therapy, mechanical traction, and exercise, and can often be healed without surgery. Unless there is a complete rupture or herniation of the disc, therapy can often get you back on your feet within a few weeks.

If however, your pain is alleviated by stretching the piriformis and flexion stretches like forward bending and pulling your knees in toward your chest, you're likely dealing with a piriformis spasm that is pinching the sciatic nerve. The piriformis attaches at the greater trochanter of the femur and the lateral border of the sacrum.

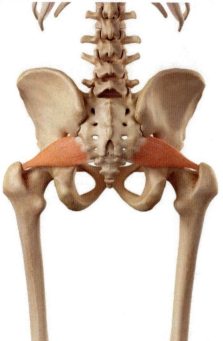

Fig. 95 Piriformis

With sitting, this muscle is put on a prolonged stretch, which over time, can result in rebound tightness, weakness, and chronic inflammation. In many individuals, the sciatic nerve runs directly through the piriformis, and for others, the sciatic nerve resides just behind it. Either way, it doesn't take much for the piriformis to cause trouble with the sciatic nerve.

Another possibility is that you are suffering from the early stages of spinal stenosis (a narrowing of the vertebral space). This can only be diagnosed through X-ray or other radiological testing, so a trip to the orthopedist is a good idea to rule this out if you have ongoing pain.

If you've had sciatica before, you know it is characterized by a deep ache in the gluteal muscles, or a sharp shooting pain down the back of the leg, and is often accompanied by some degree of numbness and tingling that can extend all the way down to the foot. Gently stretching the piriformis can be of great help and relief in this instance. Here are a few options for piriformis stretches to be done wherever you are:

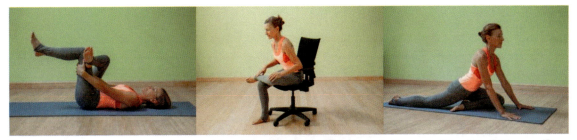

Fig. 27c Figure Four Stretch in Supine   Fig. 28 Seated Piriformis Stretch   Fig. 31b Pidgeon Pose

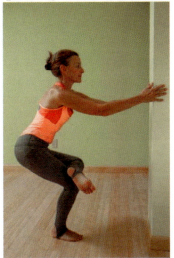

Fig. 29 Standing Piriformis Stretch

NOTE: If stretching the piriformis aggravates the condition, consult with your physician or physical therapist to rule out disc involvement or other etiology.

What often happens is that the strain on the piriformis has caused it to pull the sacrum out of alignment, which then keeps the muscle in spasm. We inherently use one side of our body more than the other and therefore, there will almost always be muscle imbalances at play. If one piriformis is weak and the other is tight, you have a perfect set up for alignment problems. In addition, if the sacral ligaments have been weakened over time due to traumatic injuries like car accidents and falls, it's no surprise that the resulting instability will create another layer of dysfunction.

This is why having a health care team is so important. Your PCP may not even look at your alignment or think of it as an issue since his/her first concern is to get you out of pain. Rest and meds are often a way to accomplish that as a short term goal. But as we discovered, meds are a temporary fix, our bodies heal faster with some amount of movement, and if we don't find the root cause of the problem, the solution—and your recovery—will remain elusive.

Look at the big picture. Consider the whole person. What's going on in your life? Is that pain in your right buttock related to an emotional stressor? An ergonomics problem? Is it that bad habit you have of carrying your wallet in your back pocket or crossing your legs? What can you do to improve the situation?

Become a problem solver. And don't stop asking questions until you get the right answers.

More pain relief

Ice vs. Heat

Rule of thumb for use of ice and heat is to use cold in the acute phase of pain (first 24-48 hours after an injury, **or to decrease inflammation**. This second caveat is important for those suffering from chronic pain due to inflammation. Ice is generally excellent for pain relief. Heat is best for relaxing tight muscles and warming the tissue before exercise or stretching, but it may aggravate inflamed tissues. Some people are very sensitive to cold and always prefer heat, while others recognize the benefits of getting beyond the icy-cold-sting of a cold pack for treating just about everything that hurts. Wrapping a warm moist towel around a cold pack before application can make it much more tolerable since the cold comes on slowly and the moisture helps with penetration. If heat is your preference, moist heat is also better than dry heat.

Our preference and tolerance for heat or cold is primarily dictated by our constitution, the unique set of qualities that make us who we are, even on a cellular level. Each individual is different, so I suggest that you try both and see which works best for you. Heat may feel nice while it's on but you may notice the muscles are throbbing and achy afterwards. This is an indicator that you may do better with a cold pack. If ice is intolerable to you for the 8-12 minutes it takes to become numb and be effective, stick to your hot pack.

NOTE: To avoid tissue injury, heat or cold should only be applied for no more than 10-20 minutes 3x per day, and you should always use layers of towel to protect exposed skin. Ice can cause burns as well as heat can. I also recommend avoiding use of electric heating pads. The body quickly adapts to the warm temperature, increasing the likelihood of leaving it on too long or falling asleep with it on, both of which can lead to deep tissue burns.

Don't forget that there are several topical pain relievers on the market. I recommend the homeopathic T-Relief for sprains, strains, and bruising. It contains a dozen herbals known for their pain reliving and healing properties. Icy Hot, Ben-Gay, and Tiger Balm are also useful, but the sensation and odor can be a bit intense. **CAUTION: Never combine topical analgesics that contain menthol with moist heat as this can cause burns.**

Chronic pain sufferers may also get great relief from the use of a home TENS (Transcutaneous Electrical Nerve Stimulation). TENS units are small, user friendly, and effective at reducing pain, inflammation, and spasm. Ask your doctor for a prescription and see your physical therapist for details. Some insurance carriers cover all or part of a trial to see if a home unit offers significant relief. You can even find them online for purchase at a reasonable price, but definitely consult with a PT to help set up the correct parameters.

If you're still having problems (muscle spasms, ROM restriction, or sciatica), you may have to look further for treatment. A PCP or an orthopedist can do special tests (X-rays, MRIs, CT scans, etc.) to rule out the possibility of disc problems, arthritic changes, and bone spurs, or other factors that may be contributing to your symptoms. But if your pain is caused by a biomechanical problem due to muscle imbalances or an alignment issue, don't expect your Western Medicine docs to be of much help, other than writing a script for meds or sending you to PT. Once you've ruled out disc problems or any other diagnostically significant conditions, you can head to your osteopath, chiropractor, PT, or massage therapist for help.

Treating Upper Extremity Conditions

Common upper extremity conditions for desk dwellers are repetitive strain injuries, most likely due to overuse and biomechanical dysfunction—known as bad posture.

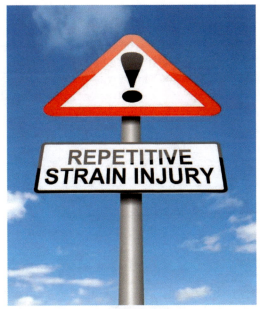

Fig. 96

- **Carpal Tunnel Syndrome** is caused by compression of the nerves coming into the hand. The problem may be coming from tightness of the retinaculum (a band of connective tissue that holds tendons in place in the wrist), or may be originating from higher up in the elbow, shoulder or neck. Nerve conduction studies are often required for correct diagnosis. Conservative treatment with physical therapy and exercise, along with eliminating contributing habits and an overhaul of the workstation is recommended. Surgery should be a last resort as it often leads to scar tissue which can cause further problems and doesn't address the root cause of the problem—which is likely biomechanical in nature. The wrist and shoulder stretches in this book can be helpful, as can a regular yoga practice to keep wrists and upper extremities strong and flexible.

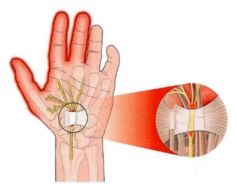

Fig. 7 Carpal Tunnel Syndrome

- **Tendonitis of the wrist extensors or flexors**, also known as tennis elbow (lateral epicondylitis) and golfer's elbow (medial epicondylitis). These debilitating injuries often come on slowly and then are aggravated by a particularly stressful physical event like a car accident, raking, gardening, washing windows, or otherwise straining the muscles beyond their already overstressed tolerance. Bracing the wrists during repetitive or resistive activities can reduce strain on the tendons that attach at the elbow, but the best way to combat this particular type of tendonitis is prevention. Stretch the wrist flexors and extensors often throughout the work day and incorporate shoulder and chest stretches to keep upper extremity muscles balanced. Full blown tendonitis can take months and sometimes up to a year to heal, even with appropriate treatment.

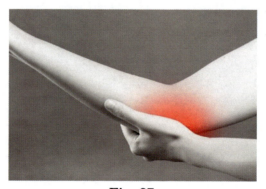

Fig. 97

- **Rotator cuff tendonitis** of the shoulder is another biomechanical and overuse issue. The job of the rotator cuff (a group of four muscles) is to internally and externally rotate the shoulder, but it is also responsible for depression of the humeral head during overhead activities, so that the tendons don't get pinched beneath the acromion process. What this means is that due to weakness and biomechanical dysfunction of the rotator cuff musculature (usually related to poor posture), the overstressed tendons become inflamed, making overhead and reaching activities painful to the point of disability. Conservative treatment of rest, physical therapy, exercise, and calming modalities like ice and anti-inflammatory medications can usually correct the problem—unless the tendons become frayed and torn as a result of repetitive strain left unchecked.

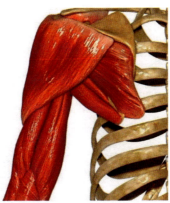

Fig. 98

- **DeQuervain's Tenosynovitis** (tendonitis of the wrist and thumb, also known as gamers/texter's thumb) **Yes. That is a real thing.** The tendon sheath around the muscles of the wrist and thumb can become inflamed with repetitive use. In addition, repetitive trauma or chronic strain can lead to arthritic changes and even ligamentous instability, in which case the tendons become inflamed due to chronically over working the muscles in an effort to stabilize the joint. Rest, ice, and limiting the offending activity are the primary recommendations.

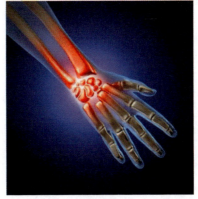

Fig. 99

Pain caused by tenosynovitis, joint degeneration, or ligamentous instability

- **Thoracic Outlet Syndrome** occurs when nerves and blood vessels coming from the neck are entrapped or compressed by tight muscles. The usual culprits are the pectoralis and scalene muscles in the front of the neck and shoulder/chest. This is often misdiagnosed as a disc problem or can easily be confused with carpal tunnel syndrome since the pain radiates into the hands and fingers. Symptoms can usually be alleviated with gentle stretches of the chest and upper extremity musculature (see the STRETCHING section of this book), massage, and physical therapy.

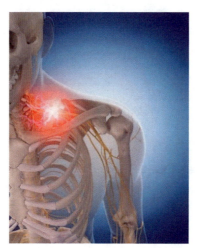

Fig. 100 Thoracic Outlet Syndrome

More tips for treatment of these inflammatory conditions.

Obviously the first step is to evaluate your workstation and eliminate contributing overuse factors as discussed in the sections on **PREVENTION** and **ERGONOMICS**. After you've adjusted your chair height, computer screen, keyboard and mouse, and limited yourself to thirty minute sprints six to eight times a day as tolerated, you'll want to add a treatment regimen.

Your first plan of attack should be to explore an anti-inflammatory diet. Certain foods like turmeric, cinnamon, cherries, berries, dark leafy greens, beans, sweet potatoes, fatty fish like salmon, and almonds all have anti-inflammatory properties. Whereas meats, dairy products (such as milk, cheese, and ice cream), hydrogenated oils, and highly processed foods are known to cause inflammation. There are several good articles and websites regarding anti-inflammatory diets on the web. Doctor Andrew Weil has some excellent information on the subject on his website. We really are what we eat, and clearly, nutrition plays a critical role in health. Why not take advantage of foods that heal? Even an increase in water, bone broths, and herbal teas can help squelch the inflammation and cleanse the digestive tract—which is the heart of the immune system. Learning which foods to eat and which to avoid is sure to improve whatever situation is causing your angst. With a bit of education, you can become your own phytonutrient pharmacist.

Beyond a nutrition overhaul and a good cleanse, massage, icing/heat, anti-inflammatory medications, gentle but consistent stretching, and acupuncture are tops on my list for treating any kind of inflammatory condition. If it doesn't improve in a few weeks, then it's off to the orthopedist or physical therapist's office. Wrist braces, Kinesio-taping, and muscle re-education can offer great benefit. Therapeutic ultrasound and electrical stimulation can also have positive effects.

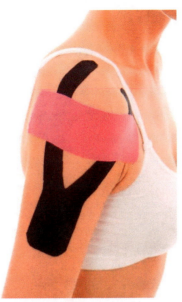

Fig. 101 Kinesio-taping to assist blood flow and offer fascial support

Another cutting edge and effective approach is Platelet Rich Plasma Therapy (PRP) that uses the healing properties of platelets taken from the person's own blood and injected back into the site of the tendonitis. Similar to this is Prolotherapy, an injection of dextrose solution into overstretched ligaments. The solution acts as an irritant, stimulating the body's natural healing mechanism and causing scarring and shortening of the ligament—a desired effect for people with chronic instability. The outcome is, typically, reduced pain and improved function, but long term results vary patient to patient. Obviously a willingness to change home and office habits, exercise, and rest as needed can determine recovery outcomes.

Other possible treatments to consider are Prolozone, Ozone, and even infrared laser treatments (known as Cold laser) which are used by osteopaths and chiropractors to treat chronic pain, inflammation, and instability with excellent results. Prolotherapy and PRP injections are done under ultrasound to locate and focus treatment on the precise area, which is different from cortisone injections, which are commonly and quite literally, hit or miss. Some site tenderness afterwards is normal with Prolotherapy and PRP but this is usually short lived. These therapies aren't covered by insurance, so it can be pricy, but I've had several clients report great enough improvement to make it worth the downsides.

Hopefully, I've given you more than enough tools to get you started on a real path to wellness. If you've tried in the past to incorporate healthy habits into your life but find your efforts short lived, stay tuned for the chapter on **MAKING AND BREAKING HABITS.** Taking control of your health is empowering, but it's also a big job. In a world where to-do lists are out of control, adding a heap of self-care responsibilities to your already overfull plate may feel like enough to put you over the edge. So before you close the book and allow your natural resistance to change to derail you before you even get out of the station, let's talk about how to manage it all and still beat the stress monster.

CHAPTER 13

STRESS MANAGEMENT 101

Since stress directly affects our health, contributes to weight gain, and is clearly a part of life we can't entirely escape, I would be remiss if I didn't discuss it here.

What is stress?

Let's start with discussing what constitutes a 'stressor,' also known as a 'challenging stimulus'. Usually, this challenging stimulus is related to an environmental condition—something happening outside of the body that requires us to adapt quickly. A stressor can be positive or negative, but in response to the stressful event, our bodies react by engaging our sympathetic nervous system, or the fight or flight response. Our adrenal glands kick in, heart rate and blood pressure soar, a cascade of hormones and neurotransmitters are released, and we go into survival mode in order to prepare for the perceived threat. Since we no longer have saber toothed tigers to worry about, a visit from Aunt Josephine can have the same effect.

Because the human body is not designed to keep this heightened state of preparedness up for long periods of time, it's the job of the parasympathetic nervous system to return our physiological conditions to normal in an effort to create homeostasis or balance in the body. When challenging conditions are ongoing—as with our hectic and non-stop lifestyles—the stress response becomes chronic and the body's ability to return to a relaxed state becomes compromised. This leads to adrenal fatigue and a host of other problems, including sleep disorders, cardiovascular disease, a weakened immune system, and anxiety and depression. Adrenaline and cortisol in high doses—two of the main stress hormones—are toxic to the body!

Good news/bad news

I once heard it said that stress is not an event; it's our response to an event. This made a lot of sense to me as each of us determines what is stress-inducing for us as individuals. What one person might consider a happy occasion—a wedding for instance—the bride and the poor person in charge of planning the event may find extremely stress inducing. There is tremendous pressure to make it the "perfect" day for the bride and groom, often leading to lots of nail biting and hair pulling for the type "A" person in charge of all the details. The expectations from others, our own expectations of ourselves, and the pressures of society to meet a certain standard combine to create a stressful situation from an event that should be a joyous occasion. Add in family dynamics and figuring out who gets to sit next to Aunt Josephine, and well…you get the picture.

One person loses their job and sees it as a terrible hardship, while another might see it as an opportunity to find something better, or a chance to return to school and get that degree they've always wanted. Having a baby can be the most wonderful experience in the world for a happy couple who have tried for years to "get pregnant," while pregnancy can be terrifying to a teenager with little family support. I think we can all agree that what is considered stressful is often a matter of perspective.

This is really good news! That means that if we can change our thinking, or reframe the way we perceive an event, we can also change our response. We all know people who seem to stroll through life smiling and letting nothing ruffle their feathers. These hardy folks seem to manage their chronic stress and still be healthy. We also know people who catastrophize every little thing and allow their health to suffer the consequences.

Now for the bad news. How we learn to cope with stressors is often the product of where we come from and how we were raised. Nervous parents create nervous children. Parents who freak out over every bump and bruise or try to "protect" their children at every turn often produce nervous, stressed out, and fearful adults. By the same token, children left to their own devices too often may be overburdened with responsibility at a young age and left feeling unsupported and chronically stressed. Each of us sees the world through a particular lens. That lens is colored by our earliest childhood experiences and how the adults in our lives taught us to react to our environment.

More good news! Fortunately, we are not doomed to accepting our parents' world view as gospel. Human beings have a tremendous capacity for adaptation. Our resilience is our superpower. That means we CAN change how we think, how we perceive the world, and how we cope with stress.

Cognitive Behavioral Therapy (CBT) is based on this principle. If we can reframe how we view a certain situation, change unhelpful thinking and behavior, and learn to see things in a different light, we can manage life's curve balls with less negative, less reactive responses. This, of course, is dependent on our willingness to change our point of view.

Stubbornness and fear will derail even our best intentions to improve the quality of our lives.

I'm convinced that there are two kinds of people. Those who will die of stubbornness and those who are too stubborn to die. I'd much rather be in the second group. I know many people who stubbornly cling to negative behaviors and make every excuse in the book as to why they "can't change." They are their own worst enemy! These are the folks who won't go to the doctor because they don't want to hear that they are overweight and have high blood pressure. They would rather stick their heads in the sand and die of a heart attack than face a reality that would require they take responsibility for their health and well-being. It's much easier to blame someone else than make real and lasting change. They blame their parents, their genetics, the world…any scapegoat will do. Down deep, they know they need to step out of their comfort zone, but the hard work involved seems overwhelming to them. Pride, blame, and fear of failure dominate their thinking and keep them resistant to making the necessary changes in their lives that would restore them to health. **Stubborn refusal to change kills more good people than any disease on the planet.** Don't let your "stinking thinking" kill you!

The other group—the too stubborn to die folks—are those who value life to the degree that they will do anything it takes to stay here on this planet for one more day. Perhaps they fear death and are clinging to this mortal coil hoping to outsmart the Grim Reaper and live forever, or maybe it's just that they see all the beauty that life has to offer and they want to stick around and enjoy it. **They know life isn't perfect, but they are determined to make every day count and to enjoy all the little miracles along the way.** This is the outlook we need to have to keep stress at bay.

Since our responses to stressors in life are basically a learned behavior based on early conditioning and whatever life experiences have colored our view of the world, it's no wonder we get stuck in old patterns and find it difficult to change. Our basic belief systems are deeply ingrained in our subconscious. We may have been shamed, abused, or made to feel unworthy as children, and those old scars keep us attached to those self-limiting beliefs. To truly make a change, we may have to go back and face those demons, cut them down, and exorcise them from our subconscious, creating new positive feedback loops that will rebuild our self-esteem.

Feeling worthy of a happy, healthy, and prosperous life is the first step to attaining it!

We must come to realize that we are no longer those impressionable children. As adults, it's up to us to choose our path. We get to decide who and what we will be, and how we will live our lives. Stress reduction, like healthy living, is a matter of choice. Retraining our thinking, doing away with old patterns of behavior, and finding new ways to cope are all within our grasp. We CAN overcome our stinking thinking—one positive choice at a time.

"The happiness of your life depends on the quality of your thoughts."—Marcus Aurelius

He also said, "You have the power over your mind, not outside events. Realize this and you will find strength."

Smart man. We can't change the people around us and we don't always have control over our environment and circumstances, but we can choose how we will respond to those things. Our mind is our own and one of the few things we can control. With practice, you'll be able to maintain your Zen, detach with love, accept those things you cannot change, and find the courage to change the things you can.

The power of affirmations

The transformative power of positive thinking, positive speech, and creating your own reality through daily affirmations are not new ideas. People like Norman Vincent Peale, Wayne Dyer, Deepak Chopra, and Eckert Tolle are experts in this area, and I highly recommend reading their books, listening to their lectures, and studying up on the subject.

A quick example of how I applied the concept of Daily Affirmations to my life:

Since I began writing toward publication in 2007, I've started every session with a few affirmations **(positive messages meant to create the reality you desire and derail the old negative thought patterns of the past).**

I say this three times:

I am an excellent writer, I am a bestselling author. Neither of these things were true when I first started on this path, but I knew it was my goal and clearly what I wanted. The first statement is now most definitely true. I feel good about my writing ability. I have several award winning young adult novels to remind me that

I'm not just full of myself (this is helpful when I hit the "I suck" part of my revisions). My skill as a writer has evolved through taking workshops, going to conferences, and studying the craft. Could it still improve? Absolutely. I've recently changed that affirmation to, **_I am an outstanding writer._** We'll see how that pans out and whether my "bestselling author" affirmation comes to fruition after I publish this book…or the next.

Perseverance and a positive attitude are the keys to success.

A few more affirmations that I have found helpful in my daily life are:

I am a money magnet.
I am happy, healthy, and whole.
I surrender to God's will for my life.
I learn something new every day.
I am a work in progress/not perfection.
I do my best at all times.
I am a positive influencer in people's lives.

Get the idea? Create your reality by speaking it into existence. Use positive, present tense language to train your brain to accept the statement as truth. Before you know it, life will start to line up with your new perception of reality. The brain is a funny thing. It can easily be tricked into believing something with enough repetition of thought. Unfortunately, we quickly admonish ourselves when we don't measure up to some externally driven expectation, and our negative self-talk takes over far too often, letting us know we'll never be good enough. I know it's easier to accept the bad stuff about ourselves, but isn't it time to rid yourself of those negative messages and self-limiting beliefs that no longer serve you?

It's time to clean out our minds like we would an old closet. Toss out the things that are unnecessary and useless, the things that don't fit, and those that make us feel bad about ourselves. With consistency and practice, you CAN unlearn self-limiting beliefs and introduce new ideas into your mind that will help you manifest what you desire.

The Serenity Prayer alone was a huge catalyst for helping me see things in a new way. Call it a prayer, or call it a mantra or meditation, it works. Once the words really sank in, I was able to develop some new coping skills to deal with whatever challenges came up.

God, grant me the serenity to accept the things I cannot change, the courage to change the things I can, and the wisdom to know the difference.

My willingness to grow and change has been the gateway to one miracle after another in my life. It has opened the door to healing in ways I never thought possible. It's not always easy—and more often than not, growth is painful. But don't let pride, stubbornness, or fear keep you from reaching your full potential and becoming your best self.

My point in sharing all of this is that I have learned to keep life's challenges in perspective and found new ways to approach stressors. **I measure everything on a brain tumor scale of life.** When stressful situations come up, I take a deep breath, find my center, and ask myself a few questions.

Can I change this situation?

If I can, and am willing to take responsibility for it, I do. If I can't, I either have to let it go, or know that if I allow it to get in my head, it will surely disturb my peace of mind. Letting go of control—or the illusion of control—and taking responsibility for those things we CAN change, is the greatest stress relief tool in our arsenal. We have no control over other people. What they do, how they feel, and how they choose to behave are not our responsibility. We can only change our responses, our attitudes, and our own behaviors. I've recently adopted the catch phrase, "Not my circus, not my monkeys." It helps me stay focused on what is truly my responsibility.

While I'm ruminating on those things that have wormed their way into my head, I ask myself this.

How does this event/situation measure up on my brain tumor scale of life?

Zero on the scale means that life is good and everyone around me is happy and healthy. Ten on the scale would mean that I, or someone I love, has been stricken with a terminal disease like a brain tumor (a worst nightmare scenario). If my problem/stressor doesn't measure more than a four on the scale, it makes it much easier to let it roll off my back. Bills I can't pay, being late for an appointment, or dealing with some idiot driver who is making rude gestures as he passes me while talking on his cell phone, are all merely a blip on the scale. I could let those things rob me of my peace of mind, or I can put them in perspective and recognize them for what they are…life's little reminders that the human condition is imperfect by nature, and that my focus needs to be on the bigger picture. This leads me to my next question.

How can I improve the quality of life for myself and others in this situation?

Taking action in a positive way empowers us. It allows us to become part of the solution rather than being part of the problem. And being a positive influencer raises our self-esteem. In keeping with my faith, it also helps me to live a life of service.

Wringing my hands won't get the bills paid. I might need to work a few more hours or find ways to work smarter not harder to increase my earnings, but I've created enough healthy relationships that I won't likely find myself living on the streets. If I use for instance, the case of my old speeding habit, I finally realized that putting myself and others at risk or getting another ticket wasn't worth rushing to an appointment to be on time. I had to choose to be aware and make a conscious effort to slow down until a new habit emerged. Also, reacting to the jerk in the car zipping past me by fuming and swearing at him won't make him less of a jerk. Sometimes, all we can do is smile and nod and stay in the moment. Meeting resistance with more resistance is where the struggle, stress, and drama comes in.

Having unrealistic expectations of ourselves and others creates unnecessary internal strife.

Reframing your perspective takes practice and effort, but once you master this principle, many of the things you once perceived as stressful become non-issues that you can easily brush off and let go. You'll find that your interactions with others are no longer fraught with conflict when you stop expecting people to behave in the way YOU think they should. I can tell you that learning to mind one's own business was no easy feat for the youngest of seven children. I still stumble into old traps on occasion, but I'm much better at recognizing them and stepping back before I fall in completely.

When I attended twelve step meetings, they used to have these cards sitting on the table with sayings like, LIVE and LET LIVE, ONE DAY at a TIME, LET GO and LET GOD. I thought at the time that these were just slogans, but seeing them every week helped them to seep into my subconscious. As I began practicing those principles, I found them to be incredibly helpful at freeing me from all the drama in my life. These simple ideas (which are anything but simple to apply, so be patient) can change the way you deal with stressors and will change your life forever.

NOTE: For another source of life changing wisdom, I highly recommend that EVERYONE (this should be required high school reading, in my opinion) pick up, read, and re-read THE FOUR AGREEMENTS, by Don Miguel Ruiz. Based on ancient Toltec wisdom, these simple precepts—when applied to our lives—are a clear path to sanity and peace. 1) Be impeccable with your word 2) Don't make any assumptions 3) Don't take anything personally 4) Do your best.

Practice these principles daily and watch the changes unfold. Adopting these new ways of thinking and being will make you feel as if you have a whole new lease on life.

How to Beat the Stress Monster

So now that you've learned to "change your mind" on the subject of stress and what constitutes a stressor, let's talk about specific tools for beating the stress monster. I call them my Army of Ms.

Massage
Enough said on the subject! Go forth and get a massage…and schedule one every month if you can. You'll be amazed at the stress reducing, health enhancing benefits.

Movement
Exercise has been shown to significantly reduce stress, anxiety, and even depression. It helps arthritis, improves cardiovascular health, lowers blood pressure, promotes restful sleep, and is the only clear path to healthy weight maintenance. Exercise also offers a boost of those lovely feel good chemicals to the brain. Endorphins are a sure-fire mood enhancer and serotonin promotes a sense of well-being. Need I say more?

Meditation (Meditation=Mindfulness)
You don't have to be a Yogi in an ashram to practice meditation. It takes only a few minutes of focused attention on your breathing to get you out of your head and into your body and to achieve a state of relaxation. Quieting the mind takes practice and consistency but is a skill that everyone can benefit from. People who meditate on

a regular basis can learn to control bodily functions such as respiration, heart rate, blood pressure, and even digestion. Meditation is calming to the central nervous system and promotes a sense of well-being. The mental benefits include clarity of thought, improved mental attitude, self-awareness, and insights that lead to personal growth. Daily practice also helps us cultivate that all-important trait of self-discipline. Even five minutes a day of deep breathing and focused internal awareness can improve your productivity and foster positivity that carries throughout your day.

NOTE: I try to meditate daily, but even if I skip a "formal" meditation practice, I'll assume mountain pose in the shower and stay there for ten deep breaths (which only takes a minute or two), all the while focusing on my breathing and how all the parts of me are working together in the pose. If you do nothing else in this book, DO THIS!

There are numerous books, YouTube videos, and meditation CDs to help you learn meditation techniques, but if you can simply find a way to spend a few minutes a day away from distractions, focus on breathing in and out, and gently coax your mind to be quiet while you take in the present moment, you are practicing a form of meditation that will offer benefits. It's helpful to create a space in your home—free of distractions—where you feel safe to decompress. Close the door, hang out the DO NOT DISTURB sign, and take ten minutes for yourself. You—and your family—will be happier and healthier for it.

Keep calm and carry on...breathe your way to peace.

If you want a more active form of meditation, you can do yoga, Tai Chi, Qi Gong, or even a walking practice where you can focus on your breath and pay attention to every movement, heal-strike, and toe-off. Notice the way your arms swing, how your feet connect to the earth, how the breath feels coming into your sinuses and filling your lungs. Take in the details of your surroundings and put it all together in a beautiful moment of connection between your mind, your body, your soul, and nature.

Prayer can have the same effect for many people, allowing them time with their Higher Power and a chance to leave the chaos behind. It's like having coffee with a trusted friend who only listens and supports you rather than trying to fix everything. You come away feeling less burdened, less alone, and stronger for having had the courage to open your heart. Whether it's a close personal relationship with God, a connection to nature, or simply a moment of self-reflection, meditation can give us the tools to stay grounded and centered, even if the world is on fire around us.

We spend so much time in our own heads and being bombarded by our devices, the constant stream of noise can be stress inducing in itself. You add the chaos of everyday life, and it's no wonder we aren't all stark raving mad! We need a time and place for recovery. Most of us don't even recognize that we have an option to step away from the madness—other than napping or spacing out on a game of Scrabble or Candy Crush. And then there's that bottle of wine we hear calling our names by mid-afternoon. (But that might just be me.) I'm not adverse to these options since they do give us a temporary respite from the clatter in our heads, but they can be a huge time suck and not very productive unless you can be disciplined about a time limit (or in regard to the wine, a calorie limit). A fifteen to twenty minute break or a power nap can have remarkable restorative properties (as can a glass of wine on occasion).

As great as those options sound, there are clearly drawbacks. **Meditation, on the other hand, supercharges our brain's recovery capacity** and is one of the best ways to maintain our sanity (and our center) amid the maelstrom our lives have become. No downside to meditating, my friends.

Meditation can take many years of practice to learn and master, but it's totally worth the time and effort. The gifts you find along the way are immeasurable. Imagine if you could simply take a breath, release it, and be in your 'happy' place amidst traffic jams, irate bosses, nagging in-laws, or hysterical teens. You might even just smile and nod when Aunt Josephine mentions how your clothes are fitting a bit snug.

Music

Music calms the savage beast. The actual phrase is *"Music has charms to soothe the savage beast,"* coined by playwright/poet William Congreve in the 17th century in his play, *The Mourning Bride*. Regardless of who said it, it's a brilliant and accurate assessment of the power of music to affect the mind, body, and emotions of every living thing. People even leave music on for their pets so Fido and Fluffy won't be so alone when Mommy and Daddy go off to work. Years ago, my husband and I did an experiment and started leaving music on for the house plants. It turned out they liked Jewel and Celine Dion, but if we played heavy metal or anything with a lot of bass or harsh beats, the plants would be wilted when we got home. No doubt, we all know that music touches a place in our souls that nothing else can, and that what we listen to is food for the soul and the psyche.

The following information is straight from the website About.com in an article on Music and Your Body: http://stress.about.com/od/tensiontamers/a/music_therapy.htm

Research has shown that music has a profound effect on your body and psyche. In fact, there's a growing field of health care known as music therapy, which uses music to heal. Those who practice music therapy are finding a benefit in using music to help cancer patients, children with ADD, and others with debilitating diseases. Even hospitals are beginning to use music and music therapy to help with pain management, to help ward off depression, to promote movement, to calm patients, to ease muscle tension, and for many other benefits that music and music therapy can bring. This is not surprising as music affects the body and mind in many powerful ways. The following are some of effects of music, which help to explain the success of music therapy:

Alters brainwaves: Research has shown that music with a strong beat can stimulate brainwaves to resonate in sync with the beat, with faster beats bringing sharper concentration and more alert thinking, and a slower tempo promoting a calm, meditative state. Also, research has found that the change in brainwave activity levels can also enable the brain to shift speeds more easily on its own as needed, which means that music can bring lasting benefits to your state of mind, even after you've stopped listening.

Breathing and Heart Rate: With alterations in brainwaves comes changes in other bodily functions. Those governed by the autonomic nervous system, such as breathing and heart rate can also be altered by the changes music can bring. This can mean slower breathing, slower heart rate, and an activation of the relaxation response, among other things. This is why music, music therapy, and sound healing can help counteract or prevent the damaging effects of chronic stress, greatly promoting not only relaxation, but health.

State of Mind: Music can also be used to bring a more positive state of mind, helping to keep depression and anxiety at bay. This can help prevent the stress response from wreaking havoc on the body and can help keep creativity and optimism levels higher.

Other Benefits: Music has been found to lower blood pressure (which can also reduce the risk of stroke and other health problems over time), boost immunity, ease muscle tension, and more. With so many benefits and such profound physical effects, it's no surprise that so many are seeing music as an important tool to help the body in staying (or becoming) healthy.

Aromatherapy

This one doesn't begin with M, but it is high on my list for reducing stress. Aromatherapy is the practice of using the natural oils extracted from flowers, bark, stems, leaves, roots, or other parts of a plant to enhance psychological and physical well-being. We all know the soothing power of walking into a house on Thanksgiving morning. The aroma of a roasting turkey, Mom's apple pie, and the mouth-watering scent of fresh baked bread can give you the feeling of being nurtured like nothing else. Who doesn't recognize and have a soft spot for the smell of chocolate chip cookies straight out of the oven? Fragrances stimulate memory, effect mood, and can help the body release toxic stress. Even if you are super fragrance sensitive—like I am—you can find natural scents that will have positive effects. Practitioners of aromatherapy are pros at finding just the right oils for treating whatever ails you. I've used lavender for great effect with treating pain and sleeplessness in children, and eucalyptus is excellent for clearing the sinuses and easing breathing problems. I'm also partial to pine, mugwort, and cinnamon.

Journaling

Also not an M word but certainly worth mentioning here as a way to decompress and reduce stress by releasing negative emotions. Writing out your thoughts and feelings can be very cathartic. It can also help you to put problems into perspective and find clarity. It doesn't have to be long and drawn out, but just putting a few thoughts onto the page—or using a voice recorder—can unburden your mind and soul. Keeping a gratitude journal is especially uplifting. Simply write down one thing you are grateful for at the end of each day. This one habit alone will make you a happier, more satisfied person. Initiate this practice with your kids before bedtime to teach them the benefits of focusing on the positive aspects of their lives.

Last words on stress reduction:
Nothing beats a balanced lifestyle for keeping stress and its effects at bay. It all comes back to the basics.

- Get adequate sleep, eat a balanced, healthy diet, exercise, and limit your exposure to stressors that you know will push your buttons. You may not be able to do this with your wayward teens, or your ornery boss, but you can do your level best to limit Aunt Josephine's visits to a few times per year.

- Staying organized is another way to combat the stress monster. A daily/weekly/monthly calendar is a must. Keep appointments and commitments under control, and whenever possible, don't overwhelm yourself. Be realistic about what you can handle and learn to say NO.

- Have no more than six items on your immediate to-do list and learn the "Brain Dump" technique of organizing. A brain dump is a complete transfer of accessible knowledge about a particular subject from your brain to some other storage medium, such as paper or your computer's hard drive. There are tutorials to teach this organizational method on the internet. It can seriously improve your productivity and organizational skill, thereby lowering your stress.

- You can't do it all and do it all well, so prioritize what is most important to you. To-do lists are super helpful, as they keep your priorities straight, and as you check off each item, you can see your progress toward meeting your goals. Don't forget to celebrate your successes, and don't be too hard on yourself about the things you DIDN'T accomplish on your list. Simply roll them into the next day. If they're still on the list weeks later, you have to re-evaluate how important the task really is, delegate to someone else, hire it out, or just DO IT.

Procrastination is fuel for the stress monster.

I discovered long ago that procrastination was more than just laziness. In many cases it's a fear of failure—which I prefer to call an attachment to failure. Attaching to or investing ourselves in the outcome of anything ultimately leads to disappointment and frustration.

Learning to detach from the outcome of things is extremely freeing. Whether we fail or succeed becomes less important than the lessons we learn from it.

Hands down, every time I'm faced with a challenging project I don't want to do, or that I feel is out of my area of expertise, it gets shoved to the back burner. I don't consider myself a lazy person at all, but when I find a particular task pushes me to learn something new or forces me to face a weakness in my abilities, I also find lots of reasons to avoid dealing with it. Old messages come to my mind, such as, *I'm not good at that, it's not my strong suit,* or my favorite, *what if…?* You fill in the blank. It's easy to get stuck on the possible negative outcomes if we fail to succeed at our task. The attachment to that success or failure is what keeps us from engaging and embracing the hard stuff.

Ruminating on *what ifs* can be paralyzing. Avoid this trap by staying in the moment and breaking the task into manageable pieces rather than trying to eat the whole elephant all at once.

We are creatures of habit and prone to take the path of least resistance, also known as, the easy way out. On an unconscious level, I tend to avoid tasks that overwhelm me or are bound to make me feel less successful. If something is perceived as "too difficult," we shrink away from it and choose to do the easier tasks or those we know we can do with a relative guarantee of success.

A wise man once said, **"Don't put off till tomorrow what you can do today."** In today's vernacular, that means, **"Get 'er done."** Or in the words of Nike, **"Just Do it!"**

Procrastination will only serve to add to your stress, since those tasks we're avoiding often "have" to be done and putting them off makes us feel like we have a weight on our shoulders like Atlas holding up the world. Simply by avoiding the task, we perceive ourselves having failed. Thus, we remain "attached to failure." If you find yourself overwhelmed with a task, ask for help or delegate it to someone who is an expert in the field. Factor into your budget ways to afford professional help or find ways to barter for services. Trying to do it all ourselves is often at the root of most of our stress. So if you can't find a way to complete the task, **say no and let it go.**

Take a breath! Don't take yourself or life too seriously. Rarely are our daily challenges a matter of life and death. We should all be grateful for that and never take it for granted. I forget who said this, but I often remind myself of the sentiment when stress starts getting me down.

"Life is too short to waste time, and too long not to have any fun."

CHAPTER 14

MAKING OR BREAKING A HABIT

Now that we've dealt with the stress monster, let's tackle those unwanted habits head on. I won't try to tell you that creating healthy habits is easy or that it will happen overnight. But it isn't impossible either. Nor is breaking an unhealthy habit. Human beings are the most adaptable creatures on the planet. Our ability to change to meet the challenges of life is one of our greatest strengths.

Before we tackle this challenging topic, I think it would be helpful to be clear about the difference between a habit, a dependency, and an addiction.

A habit is defined as a learned behavior, a settled or regular tendency or practice, especially one that is hard to give up. Biting one's nails or twirling your hair when you're nervous is a habit. Driving too fast is a habit. Talking over someone else in conversation is a habit. Habits can be broken with effort, conscious desire, and the introduction of a new stimulus that overrides the old behavior. Having a manicure on a regular basis can be a deterrent to nail biting since the nails are harder and the taste of the polish is unpleasant. Wearing hair up or keeping it short can curtail the twirling, and after a few hefty speeding tickets, it should become clear that you need to be more mindful while driving and CHOOSE to obey the speed limits. As for the talking over others in conversation, learning to be a good listener is a skill—one worth practicing and learning. It makes for better employees, friends, partners and parents.

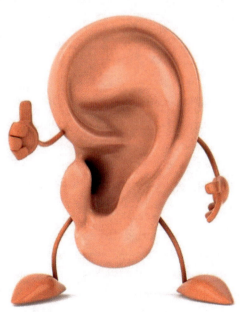

Fig. 102

Recognizing why we do the things we do is a helpful first step in overcoming bad habits, as it makes us aware of our triggers and why they affect us. Once you're aware of what triggers your response, you can work toward eliminating it or creating a new response. Creating good habits works the same way—through conscious awareness and introducing stimuli that reinforce the 'good' behavior. Then it's a matter of rinse and repeat…and repeat. **Repetition is the key to changing any behavior.**

Addiction and dependency are a bit more complicated. To differentiate the two, a simple distinction would be that a person is physically addicted to something but psychologically or emotionally dependent on something. Physical dependence in and of itself does not constitute addiction, but it often accompanies addiction.

To clarify, a number of substances produce psychological and/or emotional dependence without producing an addiction. Marijuana fits into this category. There is little evidence that pot is physically addictive, but it certainly can cause psychological and emotional dependence and become a habit that is difficult to quit because it is meeting a perceived need. By the same token, addiction can occur without physical dependence such as those with sex addiction issues, who are psychologically and emotionally addicted but not technically physically addicted to sex—although those suffering from this addiction might think otherwise. Also, physical dependence can occur without addiction, as is seen with some types of non-narcotic medications that offer such great relief from symptoms that the person is not functional without it. Dependency carries the connotation of a temporary state. A child's dependency ends with maturity. Dependency suggests a situation from which there is a way out.

Addiction, however, implies enslavement. The word derives from a Latin verb that meant, among other things, "to sell into slavery." For many years, experts believed that only alcohol and powerful drugs could cause addiction. Brain imaging technologies and more recent research, however, have shown that certain pleasurable activities, such as gambling, shopping, and sex, can also lead to addiction. Addiction exerts a long and powerful influence on the brain that manifests in three distinct ways: craving for the object of addiction, loss of control over its use, and continuing involvement with it despite harmful consequences. Addiction implies a state from which there is no escape.

An addicted person no longer belongs to himself. It is now understood that addiction is a disease, influenced by brain chemistry and even a genetic predisposition, just like Diabetes or Heart Disease. There is hope for recovery and there are effective treatments for addiction. The caveat is that the person has to be willing to admit they need help and *want* to seek treatment. **Unfortunately, the main stumbling block to recovery is often denial. The stigma attached to addiction is also a deterrent to seeking treatment, as is the complex social ramifications.**

Food addiction, for example, is a complex issue due, in part, to the simple fact that we cannot remove ourselves from the source of our addiction. We are dependent on food and we need to eat. It's like asking an alcoholic to work at a bar. Temptation and ease of access make this especially challenging for people who struggle with overeating or suffer from eating disorders like anorexia, bulimia, and binge eating disorder. In addition, there are emotional, social, and deeply rooted psychological issues attached to food addiction. There may also be biochemical factors involved that need to be addressed.

There is help and hope! Admitting you have a problem and seeking professional help is the first step. If you suffer from addiction or dependence that has you 'enslaved' and feeling helpless and hopeless,

you still have choices. You can choose to face your problem and get help today. Making that one positive choice can change your life, but you are the only one who can make it. Don't hide from the truth. Take a hard look at yourself and your life. If you aren't where you want to be, only *you* can change your circumstances. For information on addiction and recovery, check out http://www.HelpGuide.org.

Keeping these terms in mind, we are primarily talking about habitual behaviors in this text. Those behaviors that can be altered through retraining a person's thinking and a conscious choice to act differently. In contrast, dependency and addiction issues need to be dealt with by professionals in the field. Rehabilitation, psychotherapy, and recovery programs may be necessary to truly overcome negative behaviors that are jeopardizing your health and well-being. Take that step. Make a phone call. Reach out. You won't regret it.

As for making or breaking habits…

Here's the thing you need to keep in mind.

Your environment is the greatest dictator of your behavior.

If you sincerely want to make lasting changes, here is a list of to dos that may help.

- **Develop a CAN DO attitude.**

Determine what you CAN do and stop focusing on what you CAN'T DO. I've said this before, but it bears repeating. Taking responsibility and choosing to act in a positive direction is essential in breaking the habit of making excuses. Set realistic, attainable, and measurable goals. Write them down and be specific about what you want to accomplish. Start with small changes and commit to creating positive lifelong habits. It doesn't all have to happen today, but putting changes off until tomorrow is defeatist thinking. Change starts NOW! One step at a time.

For example:

Goal #1: Drink (50 ounces or however many you've determined you need) of water per day. Find a suitable water bottle and fill it right then and there, and take a sip to reinforce the new habit. Set reminders on your watch or cell phone to drink a certain number of ounces every hour if that's what it takes. Don't wait until you're thirsty. Add lemon or other fruit to flavor it if you need incentive to drink.

Goal #2: Lose a pound a week in the next three weeks. Setting short term and long term goals will help you feel less overwhelmed and make action planning easier. Action planning for this goal might include figuring out how many calories a day you need to eat and how much exercise you need to incorporate to lose that pound. Remember that one pound of fat is equal to 3500 calories. That means you have to reduce caloric intake by 500 calories per day, burn 500 more calories per day, or best case scenario, reduce calorie intake by 250 calories and burn 250 extra calories per day to add up to that pound a week. I discussed this earlier in the chapter on **FIGHTING THE BATTLE OF THE BULGE.** Choose and prepare healthy meals and grab-and-go snacks to set yourself up for success.

Goal #3: Other than work, reduce screen time by 25%. That might mean one hour less of TV, texting, or

You-tubing.

Whatever your goals are, write them down, share them with a trusted friend or family member, and commit to them. Check in often and reassess or make changes as needed. If you fall off the wagon, recommit, start fresh—NOW—and don't beat yourself up.

NOTE: Don't sabotage yourself by saying, "I'll start again on Monday." Get back in the saddle immediately. Giving yourself permission to "wait" until Monday gives a green light to your old pattern of behavior and your "excuse" thinking. You'll actually eat more that weekend knowing it's your "last hoorah," which is often the reason dieters actually gain weight while "trying" to diet. Goal setting is an art form. Be specific and frame your goals in a positive, easy to visualize format. Your words and intentions are powerful. Use them wisely.

For instance, instead of saying, "I will eat healthy today," say, "I will eat one egg, a piece of toast, and a quarter cup of cottage cheese for breakfast." You now have a concrete visual plan with a guideline you can adhere to. This works for every habit you want to create. Instead of saying "I will reduce my screen time by 25%," say, "I will shut down all household devices during this *specified time* and watch only two TV shows tonight." See what I mean? Specific, manageable, and concrete. **Visualize it and create it!**

If you truly want to reduce screen time for you and your family, set limits and stick to them by creating routines around when it's okay to use certain devices. No means no! No devices at the table should be a no-brainer, and eating in front of the TV is not the best use of family time. Two hours of screen time per day is enough for kids. Let them pick what shows they most want to watch from an approved list and monitor what games and on line activities they're engaging in.

What you feed your brain (and your soul) is as important as what you feed your body.

- **Prep for success. Clean out the old and start fresh.**

If you want to stop eating junk food, don't have it on hand. Get rid of food triggers from your pantry and refrigerator that are sure to derail your progress. Throw out the cookies, chips, ice cream, and carb-loaded processed snacks. Make yourself a grocery list that consists of nutrient dense, whole, nutritious foods, and don't shop when you're hungry. Create a manageable meal plan. Determine what you will eat for breakfast, lunch and dinner each day and plan your snacks. Stock up on simple grab-and-go foods like hard boiled eggs, pre-sliced veggies, and low fat yogurt. I dedicate an hour on Sundays to prepping foods for the week, boiling a half dozen eggs to keep in the fridge, cutting up veggies and storing them in small baggies to take to work, making serving sized containers of steel cut oats for three breakfast meals per week…you get the idea. We will always do what is easiest, so MAKE IT EASY to choose healthy.

If you honestly don't know what is good for you and what you need to avoid, educate yourself by researching "healthy foods," "nutrition for weight loss," on the internet or invest in a few sessions with a nutrition expert or dietitian. Check out my list of **snack healthy** items and **favorite smoothie recipes** at the back of this book for ideas on healthy alternatives, and visit my **PJ's Pantry page** on my website for a list of healthy foods I recommend. Since food science changes daily, I decided to keep a list that I could change as needed and revamp as new information arises, rather than listing them here.

- Initiate an exercise plan.

Even if you can't pay a personal trainer, you can start a walking routine or pick up a beginner DVD with some type of manageable exercise program. Start slow and keep it simple so you don't feel overwhelmed or push too hard too fast and injure yourself. **AVOID SELF-SABOTAGE!** If nothing else, you can incorporate the exercises I've outlined in this book. Start your good habits off for the day by **stretching** and doing your **mind sweep (see below)** before you even get out of bed and it will set you up for success for the rest of your day.

Keep your workout clothes/gym bag visible and easily accessible or dress in your workout clothes first thing in the morning. Schedule 30 minutes of exercise on your calendar at least five days per week. Shoot for three days on and one day off or every other day if this works better for your schedule. KEEP YOUR APPOINTMENT with yourself as if you have a meeting with someone important. YOU are the most important person in your life and your health and well-being MUST be your first priority. You are no good to anyone if you're unhealthy and emotionally drained. Solicit the help of friends to hold you accountable. Join a group or buddy up with a neighbor. Do whatever it takes to motivate you to be consistent.

Exercising at the same time each day will up your chances for making it a consistent part of your routine. My workouts are scheduled for 9:00 a.m. on the days I work from home, so as soon as I get up, I dress in my workout duds. No matter what I'm in the middle of, I stop at nine o'clock and get to it. My motivation is that I can't eat breakfast until I've worked out. If the clock doesn't remind me, my stomach will. A caveat is that I start my day with a few bites of cottage cheese or a spoonful of yogurt to tide me over and give my body some pre-workout fuel.

NOTE: A word on motivation. Although the example I've used here is an external motivator and might be considered a reward/punishment approach, this works for me because I also have mastered the art of creating intrinsic motivators for myself. My reason for consistent exercise goes beyond WHAT it will do for me in the short term. My reason—my WHY—is that I want to live a long, happy, productive life with my husband and be around to see my granddaughter graduate college and have kids of her own. This long term goal is at the forefront of every choice I make when it comes to my health. I am also well aware of how it feels to be strong and fit compared to being unhealthy, sluggish, and depressed about how my clothes look and feel. When I'm tempted to retreat into old habits, I revisit those feelings, pull myself up by the bootstraps, and get back on track.

To have healthy habits stick, and to overcome unhealthy habits, we need to have powerful intrinsic motivators. Consistency and a positive attitude are key.

- Try a new food.

Don't be afraid to try new foods. Spend some time at your local Whole Foods store or Farmers' Market. **Invest a small amount each week in trying a new food or healthy recipe.** Spaghetti squash is a great substitute for pasta, but if you really need some linguini, try Jerusalem artichoke pasta made by DeBoles (Jerusalem artichoke flour is derived from the tubers of a sunflower like plant), is organic, and has inulin, a pre-biotic plant fiber that helps promote the growth of healthy bacteria in your digestive system. Or satisfy that carb craving by introducing your family to the wonderfully nutritious grains, quinoa or couscous, loaded with vitamins, minerals and fiber. Add some avocado or nuts to your salads and skip the croutons. Make your own dressings. Be willing to experiment with new foods and don't let the naysayers in the family derail you. Tell them that you're doing it because you love them and ask for their support.

- **Breathe and Meditate.**

Set aside five to ten minutes a day to focus on your breathing. It can be in the shower, on a walk, or even while you're riding the bus to school or work. The idea is to be mindful about connecting your mind and body through your breath. It takes practice and discipline to quiet the mind and stay focused for even a few minutes so be patient with yourself. When your mind begins to wander, bring it back to noticing your breath. You will be amazed at the benefits of this one new habit.

- **Daily Mind Sweep**

We brush our teeth daily, bathe, and clean our homes. You'd think it was obvious that we also need to "clean our minds" from all the crap we're exposed to on a daily basis. Before you even get out of bed, do what I call a **mind sweep.** Don't lay there thinking about all you have to do that day or how you don't want to get out of bed and deal with the drudgery of your life. Don't waste time thinking about the traffic on the way to work or that meeting with your boss you've been dreading. Clear out all the negative messages by filling your mind with positive thoughts like, "Today is going to be a great day." "I'm going to rock that presentation." "I'm strong enough to handle whatever comes my way today." Don't give in to the negative Nellie in your head. Sweep her out and replace her with positive Pollyanna. Consider all that you're grateful for before your feet touch the floor. You'll find that your morning…and the rest of your day will go smoother if you do.

Marcus Aurelius said, "As you rise with the morning sun, think of what a precious privilege it is to be alive—to breathe, to think, to enjoy, to love."

- **Write down five positive affirmations.**

I discussed how to do this in the section on **STRESS MANAGEMENT.** Write your positive affirmations on fancy paper, make them pretty—a little glitter makes them eye catching—and post them everywhere. On your fridge, in your car, on your bathroom mirror. Just make sure they're visible and give you the positive boost you need to stay strong. **You are worth it!** Oooo…that's a good one.

- **Add an exercise class**.

Yoga, Pilates, Tai Chi, Qi Gong, water aerobics, or if you want something a bit more sweat inducing, try spinning or Zumba. The social aspect of organized classes can offer support and guidance as well as making you feel a sense of community and camaraderie. If the class you attend doesn't float your boat or you're being pressured to 'work harder,' don't risk your health or your self-esteem. Try a different class/studio/instructor. You're allowed to have fun. Even a once per week exercise class can offer significant benefits both physically and mentally. Twice or three times weekly is even better, but like I said before, small, manageable changes are more likely to stick. Start slow and commit.

- **Have a treat.**

Living a healthy lifestyle doesn't require you to give up everything you enjoy. If you like ice cream, cookies, or in my case…pie, have it. Once per week, limited to a serving size, and truly enjoyed (that means chewed, tasted, and then swallowed), a favorite snack won't kill you. It may even make you more determined to 'follow the rules' all week just so you can splurge on that one day. Plan the day and time of your splurge and don't allow it to turn into a binge. The same goes with alcohol. A glass of wine with dinner should be a treat, not a daily occurrence. Despite medical research touting the "benefits" of red wine, there is a tremendous amount of sugar in alcohol and it is a depressant. If you're watching your weight, or struggling with depression to begin with, save 'party' extras for weekends and special occasions. Be willing to trade off an appetizer and bread for your dessert or wine preference. You'll feel justified and rewarded for your efforts rather than guilty and regretful the next day.

I hope I haven't scared you off of eating all together. Do the best you can. Each and every healthy choice you make will have an impact on improving the quality of your life. If you've incorporated these new healthy habits, your day should look something like this:

After a solid seven to eight hours of sleep, you wake refreshed, energized, and raring to go as you do a few stretches to ease your transition from sleep to a full day of productivity. Take a couple of deep breaths before rising, set your intention to make the most of your day, and repeat the affirmations hanging on your bathroom mirror while you're staring at your reflection. Remind yourself that you are beautiful and worthy of a happy, healthy, prosperous life.

Jump in the shower, do a few more stretches and finish up with mountain pose and five to ten deep breaths. You'll be amazed at how much easier it is to deal with kids, dogs, spouses, and morning routines when you start your day this way.

Fill your water bottle first thing in the morning with plans to refill as needed to meet your daily requirement. Have a healthy breakfast (or plan it for after your workout), and plan your meals for the day, staying within your calorie limit, but allowing for snacks. Pack your food for the day if you're heading off to the office, and plan what you and the family will eat for dinner (sometimes, it won't be the same thing and planning ahead will save arguments after the dreaded question…what's for dinner?).

If you aren't an early morning exerciser, figure out where you'll fit in your thirty minute workout. This might mean bringing a change of clothes and shoes for a lunchtime hike or factoring in your visit to the gym directly after work and before you go home for dinner. If you know you won't have a spare half hour that day, plan a bike ride or walk with the kids after school, or an evening stroll after dinner with your honey.

Imagining you'll have the motivation or energy to workout at the end of the day is like saving your favorite dessert until the end of a five course meal. You might be able to do it, but you definitely won't enjoy it as much. Remember, we don't want exercise to be drudgery. Set yourself up for success by doing it early in the day and enjoying the benefits of continued calorie burn and a sense of empowerment all day long.

This goes for your meditation practice as well. If you save it for the end of the day when you're tired and just want to veg on the couch with your favorite show, it's likely not going to get done. Do it when you first get up or when you're in the shower, along with your mountain pose, or take ten or fifteen minutes of your lunch break to sit quietly and focus on your inner well-being. If this turns into a power nap, you'll still be doing yourself some good.

At work, set a timer or timer-app to remind you to get up every thirty minutes. Ignore glaring bosses and envious co-workers. If anyone says something, remind them that you are preventing injury and improving your productivity. Take a 5-10 minute stretch break and check in with your breathing, then get back to work. (This isn't an excuse to check your FB page or sports scores). Eat your lunch and snacks without consulting your cellphone, email, iPad, or other device, thereby reducing your screen time by that 25% we talked about.

Instead, try enjoying your food, chatting with a co-worker, or reading an actual physical copy of a book or magazine if your brain needs a mini-vacation from work. If you choose to work out on your lunch break, don't skip the lunch part. Starving yourself isn't the answer to healthy weight loss. Maintaining your blood sugar and 'feeding the machine' is a much more successful and tolerable approach. A lone apple is NOT lunch.

You need protein, healthy fats, whole grains, and fruits and veggies in balanced proportions to keep you going so you aren't tempted by the fast food joint or ice cream shop on the ride home. You also don't want to walk in the house starving at 6 or 7 p.m. If you work a long day, I recommend a midafternoon snack of nuts or yogurt to tide you over. I keep a bag of raw almonds in my car at all times to stave off the ride home temptations. A little healthy protein is much better for you, more satisfying, and will last longer than a jolt of coffee or a candy bar for a midday pick-me-up.

NOTE: Those of you who eat at your desk or are being "pushed" to work through lunch, remind yourself (and maybe even your boss) that you are entitled by law to a lunch break, and take it.

Once at home, prepare a healthy meal for yourself, enlisting family support in your efforts to incorporate new foods into the household diet. Don't' force this on anyone else, but definitely offer healthier options if they're willing to try them. You, yourself, know that forcing change is not the answer. People have to want to change, commit to change, and be willing to do whatever it takes to change. Having it forced upon you only makes you resentful, and those who are resenting you, even subconsciously, will do whatever they can to sabotage you. Don't fall prey to this trap. Make meal times about sharing your day and spending quality time with family. Then ask who wants to take a walk or a bike ride after dinner. If there are no takers, don't be disheartened. Go on alone or take the dog. Setting an example is the best way to affect changes in the people around you.

Wind down with some entertainment, whether that be surfing the net, playing a game with the kids, or watching an hour or two of TV, just try to stick to the time limits you've set for you and for them. Turn off electronics at least a half hour before bedtimes and end your day with a few kind words and snuggles with your loved ones. When you settle into bed, do a quick recap of all the things you did 'right' and give yourself a pat on the back. If you fell short in some areas, set your intention to do better the next day and go over an action plan in your head to achieve your goal. Doing this before you go to sleep will help solidify the plan in your subconscious.

Healthy living is about creating routines you can't live without.

CHAPTER 15

TIPS FOR SPECIAL GROUPS

In this section I'd like to offer suggestions that may be specific to your needs. The following are in no particular order, but hopefully I've covered whatever group you fall into and given you ample recommendations to help you on your way to a healthier and happier you.

The Aging Athlete

If you were like me and participated in sports most of your life, you might be starting to feel the fallout. It may be true that lifelong athletes fair better in the weight management department and naturally have a drive to be active, but they also can suffer significant degenerative joint problems because of their sports-related activities. Figure skating and martial arts were two of the toughest sports I could have chosen for my body. Repetitive trauma from falls has certainly taken its toll on my spine. Dancers and gymnasts usually fall into the category of being hypermobile and less stable in their older years (genetics also plays a part in hypermobility). Contact sports like football, hockey, or wrestling can leave bodies a bit battered and worse for wear by the time the athlete hits their forties. Most will tell you they suffer from arthritic knees, hips, shoulders, or backs. Every sport seems to have its good and bad points.

I often wish I'd known in my twenties what I know now. I might have been a little less enthusiastic in my belief that I was invincible—a common misconception among the young and fool-hearty of the world. Aging athletes need to overcome one giant hurdle in particular. In our minds we stay forever young, but as we age, we need to come to terms with the limitations of our bodies. Making the choice to reduce or eliminate high impact activities, replacing them with something less traumatic on our joints, is like asking junk food junkies to limit themselves to sprouts. It goes against our grain to accept defeat, throw in the towel, and take up the yoga mat in place of the martial arts mat. A lucky few are able to keep running and cycling well into their seventies and eighties, but for most of us, we likely need to tone down our activities to less impactful sports.

Water aerobics, swimming, light weight training, gentle yoga, Pilates, Tai Chi, or Qi Gong are all excellent options for arthritis sufferers or those who are attempting to save their bodies from further damage. Just remember that the goal is to keep moving. Treat your chronic pain issues as outlined earlier in the book, and consult your physician about prescription pain medications if your pain becomes unmanageable, but be wary of opioid addiction if you're treating an ongoing chronic problem. Employ alternative therapies for pain management like acupuncture, massage, and energy work. Joint replacement may be an eventuality, but take heart—technology has come a long way and is making strides every day in state-of-the-art care for partial and total joint replacements.

Do the research, talk to your doctor, and decide what's right for you. Listen to your gut about what your body needs and commit to taking care of it.

The Weekend Warrior

Are you one of those people who sits at a desk all week and when Saturday rolls around decides to ride your bicycle 50 miles, hike a mountain, or slap a roof on the house? Do you try to fit a week's worth of activity into two days? Granted, we all try to pack our time off with chores that need doing or fun time with the kids, but if we go from zero to seventy between Friday and Monday, we're likely going to encounter some resistance from our bodies.

The answer, of course, is balance. Add more movement into your work week and more rest time on the weekends. It shouldn't be all or none in either case. I rotate my workout days with the goal of three days on and one day off of my hard-core thirty minute routine and then repeat. This gives me a pretty good guarantee that I'll get at least four or five days per week of consistent exercise. I add walks, yoga, and an occasional kayak excursion to keep it fresh and fun. I also try to ensure that one of my days off lands on the weekend so I can really have a day of rest. During the work week, try to fit in at least three days of exercise, so that when the weekend rolls around, you haven't been sitting on your butt for five days straight. This doesn't bode well for then being super active. Going from nothing to too much is NOT healthy and increases your risk of injury.

At the very least, consider yourself a domestic athlete and do a bit of warm up and stretching before you tackle four hours of lawn work or gardening on Saturday morning. Stop and take stretch breaks, drink plenty of fluids, and remember to stretch afterwards as well. Incorporate dynamic stretching into playtime with the kids (think toe touches, alternating lunges, or arm circles with a military march—which works coordination as well as flexibility. Kids love to do downward facing dog). You'll be both setting a good example and prepping your body before tossing/ batting/ or kicking the ball around.

Adopting the simple tips above can significantly reduce soreness and risk of injury.

Rabid Readers

Along with writers, desk dwellers, and gamers, avid readers have a hard time balancing their sitting life and their moving life. If you've ever engrossed yourself in a page turner, you know how hard it is to stop and put the book down. Reading is such a wonderful escape from the routine of our own lives, the temptation to slip into another world and someone else's head for a few hours is simply too great to resist. There are also those people who must read for a living. Agents, editors, proofreaders and such, spend hours a day pouring over novels, while corporate types and attorneys spend much of their day looking over briefs and contracts. Hobbyists may have more flexibility with their time, but some are prone to devour five to ten books a week, ignoring their screaming necks and their ever widening backsides.

PJ's Top Five Tips for Readers:

1) Find a comfortable, ergonomically supported place to read. Don't get sucked in by the couch monster where you'll find yourself sitting folded into a ball in the corner, your neck and back in agony at the end of an hour. Use pillow supports to keep you upright and rest your arms over a few pillows in your lap to support the book so it's at eye level.

2) Read in sprints. As I suggested for your computer/screen time, set a limit on your reading time. Commit to moving for at least ten minutes every few chapters or every thirty minutes—whichever comes first.
3) Switch to audiobooks. Or at least alternate between print, digital and audio. The variety will broaden your experience as well as giving you the flexibility to get your brain candy while you're doing your housework, exercising, or even walking on the treadmill. Most treadmills have a shelf for your e-reader these days.
4) Drink plenty of water (always have a water bottle nearby and refill as needed). This will force you to take bathroom breaks and discourage snacking.
5) Snack healthy. Many readers love to snack as part of their "escape" mentality. The problem—beyond the unhealthy choices we make—is that we are so into our stories that we aren't mindful about the quantity or quality of the foods we are putting into our bodies. Choose low calorie, nutrient dense snacks such as almonds, carrots, or apple slices rather than chips, chocolate, or ice cream. Pay attention to serving sizes and only have that amount on hand as you read.

Make these conscious choices ahead of time so you don't fall prey to mindless eating or succumb to the couch monster.

Couch Connoisseurs

I prefer this term to couch potato, a throwback phrase coined in the '70s to describe a person who lounged about and purportedly watched too much television. It has the connotation of laziness that I don't particularly care for, so let's reframe that and consider ourselves *couch connoisseurs*. We know how to relax and we're proud of it! If I've worked hard all day and need some much deserved down time, escaping into a few action shows or watching something that makes me laugh is a welcome—and dare I say—healthy distraction. Until it's not. If I allow myself to vegetate there for the next four hours, I'm not only wasting an incredible amount of time on mindless entertainment and therefore missing out on "real life," I'm also contributing to my Sedentary Lifestyle Syndrome and all that comes with it. Pick and choose how and where you want to spend your entertainment hours, and adhere to screen time limits as if your life depends upon it. I have a feeling that ultimately, it does.

I mentioned the couch monster above. We have all found ourselves parked on the couch for hours at a time. I'm not immune to gorging on *Walking Dead* marathons or catching back to back episodes of *Game of Thrones*. But the rules still apply. Set limits, get up and move every half hour, hydrate, and snack healthy. Use good ergonomics, support your body as needed, and practice your self-massage techniques to keep your muscles happy and your blood circulating. Invest in quality furniture or at the very least, use firm pillow supports and don't let the couch inhale you, further contributing to rounded shoulder/forward head posture.

The Techno-Teen

If you're a teenager and you're reading this book, FANTASTIC! Forewarned is forearmed and you're still in the early stages of your sitting career. Now is the time to create good habits and learn to combat the signs and symptoms of SLS. The longer you live with habits, the harder they can be to change. One recent study showed that two out of three teens are now spending more time on their devices than they are sleeping. That can't be good!

No doubt, you're already having issues with muscle imbalances that are making good posture a challenge. By nature, teens are slouchers. Don't take it personally. I believe this is due to a desire to "hide" from unwanted attention when they're going through that awkward phase of puberty. As much as teenagers want to assert their independence and be different, the pressure to fit in is extraordinary, and the mentality that *if you aren't in your out,* prevails. Tall kids, especially, will be prone to rounding their shoulders and slumping in an effort to "fit in" with the crowd. The result is chronic muscle imbalance and all the orthopedic problems that come with it that I've described in this book. Even if you hate hearing it, you're mom is doing you a favor by reminding you to sit up straight.

You might also be suffering from signs of gamer's/texter's thumb, characterized by a pain in the tendons along the thumb side of your wrist. The solution seems simple enough. Limit or discontinue the activity that is causing the problem. Since most teens would rather have an arm cut off than give up their tech devices, the solution—although simple—is not so easy. If the condition goes untreated and becomes chronic, it can really put a person out of commission. It would make writing, gripping, lifting, carrying, or even zipping up your pants, difficult. That's a high price to pay for ignoring the early signs of this form of tendonitis. Is Angry Birds or Mine Craft really worth it?

Perhaps you're beginning to notice headaches, fatigue, and weight management issues. Whether you want to admit it or not, excessive screen time is the problem. Your parents may have already set limits around how much TV time or gaming/tablet time you're allowed, but they can't watch you every second of the day. We both know your life revolves around technology, and that given an inch, you'll take a mile. That's why it's up to you to set your own limits.

You aren't a little kid anymore and your parents can only do so much to guide you. They themselves are probably struggling with their own screen time issues and may not be setting a perfect example. Technology entertainment and communication is as tempting for them as it is for you and tech addiction is no joke. It can take hold of anyone. Maybe it's up to you to set the standard—or at the very least—work with them on it. I know it isn't your job to teach your parents about healthy habits, but I can tell you, they will appreciate your enthusiasm and cooperation more than you know.

After all, your generation is the one that will have to deal with the fallout of how we manage this problem today. Unless you take control of maintaining your health as society adapts to this digital age, society as a whole will suffer the consequences. Obesity is reaching epidemic proportions, degenerative conditions of the musculoskeletal system are at an all-time high, and we still don't know the long-term radiological effects of over-exposure to all of our electronic gadgetry. It is definitely effecting the way we communicate—or don't—and how we interact with the world around us.

Lack of eye contact, fear of casual touch, and avoidance of face to face interaction is the new norm as we text our way through life and keep our noses buried in our cell phones. Ironically, in our efforts to connect with the world, we are losing our personal connection to each other. The more personal distance we create between us and those closest to us, and the more we inundate ourselves with negative messages and violent images in the media, the more isolated and antisocial we become.

Over time, this can have dramatic emotional effects. As humans, we thrive on direct relationships with one another and depend upon each other for emotional support—and dare I say, even our very survival. Making meaningful and necessary connections are what make us human at our core. Are we in danger of losing our humanity to technology? I hope not. Time will tell, and it's likely that you, generation Z, will determine the fate of humanity. It's an awesome and terrifying responsibility, but I have faith that you are up to the task. I understand the social pressure to participate in what's popular, and the constant reminders that we'll never measure up to the world's standards of perfection. The need to belong is a powerful driving force, but **the person who changes the world is the one who stands up when everyone else is sitting down.**

Be the change!

I challenge you to keep track of your screen time for one week. How much time are you spending watching TV, talking/texting on your cell phone, checking out YouTube, or gaming? I imagine that the number of hours per week will blow your mind. According to the Kaiser Family Foundation, teens are spending upwards of seven hours per day and fifty hours per week watching TV and using electronic devices.

So my first suggestion is to treat texting and gaming as a sport. I know it sounds crazy, but seriously, I know there are "texters" out there who move their thumbs across that keypad at warp speed. I personally, have the manual dexterity and hand-eye coordination of a three-toed sloth, but kids today are practically born with a controller in their hands.

PJ's Top Ten Tips for Techno-Teens:

1) **Warm up.** It may seem ridiculous, but it will help, trust me. Shake your hands, wiggle your fingers, and do some shoulder rolls and neck stretches before engaging in your techno-athletic event.
2) **Watch your posture.** Ergonomics isn't just for the corporate world. Everyone has a PC and spends far too many hours in a seated, slouched, and sedentary position. This is something you can change and control. It might take some effort and cost a few bucks to get the optimum setup, but it's worth it to save yourself and your body the long term problems.
3) **Moderation.** Take frequent breaks, change positions, and rest your poor over-stressed thumbs. Set limits for yourself and create habits around those limits to help you stay on track. (i.e.: Full water bottle=frequent bathroom breaks and an opportunity to stretch.)
4) **Oh yeah, STRETCH!** Check out some of the stretches in this book and incorporate the ones that suit your needs. The wrist/forearm/shoulder stretches are especially helpful and can be done even while you're sitting at your desk in school.
5) **Be social.** See friends and plan activities in a group at least once or twice a week. Bonus points for planning a hike, a bike ride, or other physical activity—preferably one that's parent approved.
6) **Eat dinner away from the TV** and commit to a "Tech-free zone" at the table.
7) **Turn off/silence** your phone, computer, and other devices at least thirty minutes before bed. **(It helps to have a centralized charging station for phones and tablets so parents and kids both**

know where gadgets belong at bed time and you won't have "forgotten" to charge your electronics for the next day.)

8) **Record your favorite shows** so you can watch them at a convenient time that won't interfere with homework and appropriate bed times. This will also save you watching the million commercials advertising fast foods sure to increase your waistline.

9) **Spend a few minutes of quiet time** with yourself every day. This might consist of prayer, meditation, journaling, or just lying on your back staring at the clouds on a sunny afternoon. There seems to be some misconception that human beings have to be doing something at all times. It's really okay—and quite healthy—to just "be." Revel in these moments of quiet reflection. Try not to dwell on negative emotions, but instead, take a few minutes every day to think about what you're grateful for. Counting your blessings is the quickest way to put life into perspective and keep you grounded in positive thinking. No electronics required.

Remember; you are a human being…NOT a human doing.

10) **DON'T TEXT AND DRIVE!** You're probably sick of hearing this, but cell phone use while driving is a public safety hazard that is out of control. Texting while driving is now the leading cause of death for teen drivers, surpassing drunk driving. About 3,000 teens die annually and 300,000 are injured in automobile accidents caused by cell phone use while at the wheel. Don't be a casualty. Turn off your phone when you get in the car, leave it in the back seat, glove compartment, or trunk, or simply don't answer it. NOTHING is so important that it can't wait until you have reached your destination. If it is that important, pull over and park the vehicle to take the call.

NOTE: Most cars these days have Bluetooth compatibility and allow for hands free communication. If your vehicle doesn't have this feature or you are, at any time, caught with your hands on a phone, you will get ticketed in most states. Don't risk losing your license…or your life.

Tips for kids, tots, and toddlers

We often think of small children as energizer bunnies. They seem to have boundless energy and are constantly on the move. But even with today's hectic lifestyles, childhood obesity has more than doubled in children and quadrupled in adolescents in the past 30 years. The percentage of children aged 6–11 years old in the United States who were obese increased from 7% in 1980 to nearly 18% in 2012. The numbers are leveling off, but clearly, there is still a problem. So what's happening to our kids?

Children are faced with the same challenges as adults when it comes to eating healthy and getting enough activity in this digital age where screen time is a huge part of their lives and they're becoming more and more sedentary. But not only do children not have control over their diets or their exposure to what ails society, we adults are setting a bad example. If we don't set limits around screen time for ourselves and don't take time to prepare healthy, balanced meals, our children will suffer. The best gift you can give your child—besides your love and attention—is the gift of lifelong healthy habits. Here are a few suggestions for keeping your tots, toddlers, and pre-teens healthy, happy, and fit.

- **Set up scheduled exercise times.** I suggest that after school, rather than forcing kids to sit down and do homework right away (since they've already spent their entire day sitting), that you initiate some form of physical activity. Avoid the trap of allowing them to park in front of the TV or entertain themselves with electronic devices for hours on end. If they aren't already involved in sports, sign them up for intramurals, local park and recreation activities, or simply start a neighborhood play group. Ask a few moms/dads to take turns hosting one day a week. There are some great Yoga for Kids and exercise DVDs available for rainy days and plenty of ways to create active play for children. Even toddlers can be taught the virtues of downward facing dog and I haven't met a kid who doesn't love Simon Says…take three hops forward. You fill in the activity.

- **Healthy snacks** are a must. I'm convinced that sugary, highly processed foods are at the root of many behavior problems, including ADD and ADHD, as well as the childhood obesity epidemic. Studies show that hyperactivity disorders and attention deficit symptoms improve with reducing the intake of refined sugars and processed foods. Limit candy and refined sugars and completely eliminate soda from your child's diet. They need to be hydrating with pure, clean water just as much as adults do—if not more so. (Serve filtered water whenever possible.) Watch out for hidden sugars in foods such as breakfast cereals, juices, and white flour products like white breads, cookies, and baked goods. Stick to whole food snacks like fruits, vegetables, high fiber, high protein and whole grain products. See my section on **HEALTHY SNACKS** for more ideas.

- **Limit screen time.** I know I'm repeating myself again, but I'm amazed at how babies seem to come into the world knowing the ins and outs of technology. They are just as fascinated by it as adults and teens. The draw of instant gratification and perceived control over their external universe has a strong pull. High resolution graphics and bright colors are highly attractive to the human eye. But as fun as it may be, it should be clear by now that there are negative consequences to overexposure to technology. By allowing excessive screen time—even if it's educational—we are setting our children and toddlers up for a sedentary lifestyle and a host of bad habits. We must make the choice for them and set limits for computers, tablets, and television time. That includes having them in the room when we're watching our favorite shows. Even if it seems they aren't paying attention to what we watch, they are receiving the messages. Avoid watching violent, over sexualized, or graphic content with the kids around. Even watching the news can be stress-inducing for children. DVR your favorite shows and watch after kids are in bed. Limit their TV viewing to age appropriate programming and strictly adhere to time limits of two hours or less of total screen time. There are far more constructive and creative activities to occupy their time.

- **Cultivate creativity.** Since many school systems are struggling with budgets and core curriculum requirements, programs like art, music, and physical education are falling by the wayside. It's now in the hands of parents to provide these more creative and physical pursuits to produce a well-rounded education for their children. Studies have shown that kids who learn music or play instruments do better in math, and that art in all forms, cultivates self-expression and builds self-esteem. In addition, proper education in physical fitness is essential for healthy development and growth. If we want our children to develop a lifelong appreciation for exercise and healthy lifestyle habits, we need to promote fitness and help them develop an *exercise is fun* mentality.

- **Teach kids to breathe and meditate.** Even small children and toddlers can be taught to meditate. This may seem a bit over the top if you don't have a meditation practice of your own, but you can instill a lifelong habit in your children that will benefit them in ways you can't even imagine. Commit to learning together. Simply spending a few minutes before bed practicing progressive relaxation exercises can improve the quality of their sleep and teach them to calm themselves after a full day of dealing with the challenges of life. If they learn to take deep breaths and focus on the sensations in their bodies as they contract and relax each muscle group, they will learn invaluable life skills for coping with stress. They will be more self-aware and able to deal with negative situations in a positive way. Play soothing music at night and read with your children often. Not only will you be nurturing their personal growth and development, you'll be creating positive experiences they will hopefully pass along to their own children.

- **Family time and one on one contact.** I know it's challenging to carve time out of your day for all the minutia like getting kids to brush their teeth, eat, dress, and find their shoes, let alone spending one on one time with them—especially if you have a brood, a job, and are trying to find a minute to take care of yourself. But here's the thing. They grow up incredibly fast, and every minute that you spend with them will seem all the more precious to you—and to them—when they are no longer under your roof. You only get one chance to give your kids a great childhood.

> **Make time every day to check in with how they are doing. Whatever is important to them, make it important to you. Read, sing, dance. Play games, build forts, talk. Stop yelling and try whispering. Breathe. Hug. Snuggle. Teach them to love life, nurture nature, and embrace empathy.**
> **You'll never regret it.**

Injured or Infirmed?

Despite our best efforts and greatest desires to be healthy and active, the Universe sometimes throws us a curveball. An accident, injury, or illness can knock us down out of nowhere or creep up on us over time, robbing us of our sense of security, our independence, and even our livelihoods. I get it. You're in pain, you may not be able to work, bills are piling up, and your family, though kind and patient with you, are wondering where their source of constant love and support has gone and when he/she will return. It's hard to be chipper when life is sucking. It's also difficult to find the motivation to do anything about it.

Depression often follows on the heels of an injury or illness. We fear we will never get better, or that we'll have to live with the limitations and pain we are currently experiencing. A sense of hopelessness seeps in. This will often lead to a downward spiral and attempts to self-medicate with alcohol, drugs, or food—a triple whammy to avoid if possible, as it will only exacerbate your problems in the long run. You may be on pain meds prescribed by your doctor, but this can quickly become a nightmare scenario if you have a predisposition to addictive behavior or the meds aren't managed properly. Short term use of prescription pain drugs is perfectly acceptable in the acute phase of recovery, but if you're still on them six weeks later, you're likely to run into trouble with the vicious cycle of a self-perpetuating pain loop and opioid addiction. Your body will begin to send pain signals when the meds wear off because your brain is now trained to expect the drug.

There are better solutions. First, let me say, it's been my experience in life that nothing lasts forever. Life is constantly changing, adapting, and evolving. You will too. Your body wants to heal itself, and given the right tools, it can. I won't promise a full recovery (degenerative diseases are called that for a reason), but I can promise that if you follow these suggestions, the quality of your life will be better for it.

NOTE: Consult your physician before discontinuing any medications.

Tips for the "Forced-To-Be-Sedentary"

- **Believe you can get better.** A positive mental attitude is your #1 defense against chronic illness and becoming debilitated. It goes back to cultivating that CAN-DO attitude, focusing on what you can do and not what you can't.
- **ISOMETRICS**—Almost anyone can do isometric exercises, no matter how infirmed they are. Tighten, hold, breathe, and relax three to five times for every muscle group in your body that DOESN'T hurt. This is also how we do **progressive relaxation exercises**, which are great for calming the mind and helping the body relax. Assume your best posture and start with squeezing the major muscle groups like the glutes (glut sets), and abdominals (tummy tucks). Work your way down your legs to your feet, contracting and relaxing each muscle. It takes some time and focused attention, but that's the beauty of PRE's. Without getting out of bed or your favorite overstuffed chair, you're increasing your circulation, engaging your mind in a positive activity, and strengthening in a safe, gentle way. One might even call this a meditative experience. It gets you out of your "pain brain" (where all you can think about is how much pain you're in), and focused on the "healthy" parts of your body. It also brings awareness to the breath, thereby decreasing your heart rate, blood pressure, and stress level.

   When you've completed the lower extremity isometrics, move on to your arms, making a tight fist, contracting your biceps—whatever muscles are working—work them! Trust me. It's a workout even if you're bed-ridden or stuck sitting on the couch for six weeks with a cast. Isometrics are also great for helping maintain strength of stabilizing muscles that will become necessary when you're up and about.
- **Stretching** helps blood flow, relieves muscle tension, and reduces pain. Find the stretches you CAN do, and do them. Any amount of movement is going to improve the situation. Yoga can be done in a chair and there are more and more classes like this offered at senior centers. Don't get hung up on the age requirements. Seniors can be a great source of inspiration, wisdom, comfort and companionship during a long recovery process, so don't rule out programs designed for the elderly if you are currently debilitated. They love spending time with "young people" and will welcome you with open arms.
- **Aquatic Therapy**—I highly recommend aqua therapy for anyone suffering a debilitating disease or injury. Because of two properties of water—buoyancy and hydrostatic pressure—an aquatic environment is the perfect medium for gentle, low impact exercise. Improve flexibility, strength, muscle endurance, and stability with a healing modality that has been used for millennia.
- **Get support/ask for help**—If you're like most people, you're happy to lend a helping hand when someone you love is sick or injured, but you hate asking for it for yourself.

Why do most of us feel guilty asking for help, and why on earth do we feel undeserving of support? Needing help when you're sick or hurt is not weakness—it's a simple fact of life and a byproduct of being human. As part of the life cycle of every being, we all must submit to our own mortality and frailty at some point in our lives. The trick is handling these times with grace, dignity, and integrity.

Vulnerability raises an innate fear response within us (since we'd rather not be prey to any saber-toothed tigers while we're laid up). The last thing we want to do is be a burden to our families.

Stop allowing pride, fear, and guilt to rule you.

- **REFRAME your thinking.** Try to focus on what you can learn through the situation and how you can make the experience positive for everyone involved by being a cooperative patient with a positive outlook.

Pride, fear, and guilt are highly motivating forces—but not in a good way. Fear of failing our loved ones or being permanently disabled can set us on a path leading straight to depression.

I'll add here that stubborn refusal to ask for help is only beneficial if it pushes you toward independence and doesn't leave you feeling resentful. The people in your life can't read your mind. If you don't ask, they may not know what you need from them or how they can help. I'm not saying you should be waited on hand and foot—although that might be necessary in the short term—but don't let your stubbornness derail your recovery by doing too much too soon. Delegate chores you know are beyond your capabilities and make a honey-do list with the three top priorities in bold so everyone knows how best to help you, but don't take it personally if not everything gets done. In addition to teaching us to be patient and compassionate with others, needing help humbles us—a state I'm convinced has many lessons to be learned and benefits to be had.

A NOTE TO CARE GIVERS: If you need to hire help, hire help. You may have to do some creative financing, enlist the help of reluctant family members, and/or track down every agency and insurance plan that might offer assistance, but it will be worth the effort to have even one or two days off per week to live your own life. You need to maintain your autonomy and re-fill the well or you'll have nothing to give to your loved one.

Whether you are injured or infirmed, an aging athlete, a weekend warrior, rabid reader, couch connoisseur, techno-teen, toddler or tween, I hope you've found some useful advice in this book. Whatever category you fall into, make your health your #1 priority, thereby setting an example for those around you and ensuring that you and your family have many happy, healthy years ahead.

CHAPTER 16

PJ'S SNACK HEALTHY TIPS & SMOOTHIE RECIPES

Snack Healthy Tips

The following are only a few suggestions for snacking healthy and creating some nutritious and delicious smoothies. I encourage you to explore, experiment, and load up on healthy goodies. As you've seen, I'm a fan of feeding the machine. Keeping your blood sugar level throughout the day is essential to maintaining a healthy metabolism, and requires that you eat about every 3-4 hours. If you're one of those people who only eats one or two big meals per day and then laments the fact that you can't lose weight, this especially goes for you. It's been shown that grazers do better than big meal eaters when it comes to weight maintenance. Mainly because of how each style of eating effects hormonal balance and metabolism.

The trick is to keep meals and snacks to appropriate calorie counts, serving sizes, and nutritional values based on your daily dietary needs. In other words, divide up your daily calorie allowance into three larger meals and two snacks per day, and consider how you'll get your fruits, veggies, meats, grains, and dairy into your diet.

For example, and we'll make it easy; say you have a 2000 calorie per day allowance in order to maintain your current weight. (See my chapter on **Fighting the Battle of the Bulge** to determine your daily requirement). You'll want to plan your breakfast, lunch and dinner to contain about 500 calories each and have two snacks per day of 250 calories. Feel free to have less for breakfast and more for lunch or spread the calories out the way you'd like, but try not to load too many onto one meal. Two thousand calories is a lot of food. Spreading the calorie load evenly like this throughout the day is so much better for you than having two one-thousand calorie meals that cause your blood sugar to spike and later crash, leaving you feeling listless, fatigued, and depressed. So figure out your calories, choose nutrient dense foods, and snack away two times a day!

Here are my picks for healthy, nutritious snacks that will fuel your mind, body, and soul, giving you the foundation you need to stay on top of your game, and help you put your best foot forward all day. The following are all 250 calories or less.

Almond butter and…apples, celery, carrots, or a half a banana. Really, almond butter on anything is pretty great. Try a variety of nut and seed butters for their high protein content and healthy fats (just pay attention to serving sizes). Choose organic if possible and avoid any that have added ingredients like sugars and stabilizers. Other than nuts and a little salt, you shouldn't see anything else listed on the label. Make your own, buy it fresh at your local whole foods, or find it in a health food store. Health food stores can be pricey so shop around. I actually buy mine at Costco and stock up for a very reasonable price. Prices are subject to change depending on yield of global crops. Almonds require a considerable amount of water to grow, and drought conditions in the Western U.S. are having an impact. Remember, other nut and seed butters may be used as a substitute, so experiment. I prep my fruits or veggies and store them in small plastic containers, then I take a separate small container of nut butter and use it to dip the snack into. Two tablespoons is a serving size and around 200 calories. I use a single tablespoon to cut the fat and calories in half and make up the other 100-150 calories in the fruits or veggies department.

Hard Boiled Eggs are a great grab-and-go snack. I cook up a batch on Sundays and have them throughout the week for snacks, sandwiches, and in salads. I buy organic here for humanitarian reasons as much as for the health benefit. Short of raising them myself (which I've done and plan to do again soon), this is the only way I know that the source of my eggs—quirky and fun-loving chickens—are treated humanely, not pumped full of antibiotics, and are fed only organic feeds without pesticides, drugs, antibiotics or animal byproducts. Well worth the extra cost in my opinion. A single egg has only about 72 calories and boasts an energy boosting, muscle building 6.3 grams of protein. Eggs are a significant source of cholesterol (about 186 mg), but the latest research shows that eggs are not as bad for us as they once believed. The 4-5 grams of fat in an egg is nicely divided between saturated, monounsaturated and polyunsaturated fats, putting it on the "good fats" list, or at least on the "not so bad for you" list. In moderation (no more than six a week), eggs—hardboiled, poached, or used for baking—are back on the menu!

Yogurt is another high protein snack that gets my vote for satisfying my energy and taste needs. **But not all yogurts are created equal.** Most are high in sugar, and even some organic yogurts have considerable sugar added. Buy the plain yogurt and add your own fruit and sweetener if needed to control the sugar content. An added tablespoon of ground flax seed will add fiber and a healthy dose of plant omega-3. Or you can have plain Greek yogurt with slivered almonds, a dash of vanilla and a pinch of cinnamon. Yum!

NOTE: Yogurt makers are becoming more and more popular. It's a fun, easy project to do at home with kids, and you can control what's added. With a little experimentation and practice, you can be your own yogurt aficionado!

Veggies and dip are always tasty, satisfyingly crunchy, and super nutrient dense. I make my dip with plain Greek yogurt, adding dill or fancying it up with some herbs or spices. Hummus (made from ground chick peas, sesame tahini, and garlic) is another high fiber yummy alternative to traditional dips. You can also create your own creamy avocado dip by mixing an avocado with plain Greek yogurt, a bit of lime or lemon juice, minced cilantro (if you like), and a dash of cumin, salt, and hot pepper sauce to taste if you want something spicy. Carrots, celery, or just about any kind of raw veggie works with this.

Apple sauce and cinnamon offers an easy option if you're looking to satisfy a sweet tooth. I buy organic, no sugar added apple sauce. Just a pinch of cinnamon adds an apple pie-like flavor. 1 cup tops out at under 150 calories.

Dipped strawberries or bananas are a special treat and reserved for when my chocolate demon won't be silenced. Melt down 2 squares of dark chocolate, dip 1 inch slices of banana or 5 strawberries half way into the melted chocolate and place them on a plate in the fridge (use toothpicks). An hour later, you've got a decadent dessert or a late afternoon craving fix.

Dehydrated fruit and/or homemade trail mix works great for school lunch boxes and snacks for the ride home from work to keep you out of trouble. Dehydrators are fun and easy, are versatile, and a must for every pantry. If you don't have one, or don't have the space for one (they are a bit cumbersome), you can use your oven set on the lowest temperature. Line the bottom of the oven with foil to catch drips and leave the door open an inch to let moisture escape.

Clean, peel, cut, and thinly slice just about any kind of fruit (the thinner the better, as thicker pieces will take longer). Dehydrators come with several "racks," so do as many varieties of fruit as you like. Usually you'll need to dehydrate them for several hours. Follow the instructions that come with your dehydrator or search the web for recipes and specifics for dehydration times for each fruit. The more natural juice a fruit contains, the longer it will take to dehydrate. You'll want to experiment a bit to decide on the best thickness and time for each. Once you have it down, you'll have a variety of sweet, tangy options for snack foods. Hard or firm fruits like apples, pears, and bananas make nice "chips," while strawberries, pineapple, peaches, or mango take longer and are best sliced thinly. You'll still have a sweet, chewy snack that packs a flavor explosion. Do eat dried fruits in small, serving size quantities as they are high in natural sugars.

You can even make a paste of your fruit, spread it thinly, dehydrate it and make your own fruit roll ups. Once dehydrated, cut some of your fruit into smaller pieces and mix with granola/nuts/and a handful of dark semi-sweet chocolate chips. Divide into small serving size baggies so you won't be tempted to eat too much. This is nutrient dense, but also high in calories. A ½ cup serving will be about 200 calories.

NOTE: The dehydrator also makes fantastic turkey jerky—a great high protein hiking snack. Since I marinate my turkey strips in organic soy sauce and Worcestershire sauce, along with a few other spices, they do have a high salt content, but if I'm hiking and sweating, this is a nice way to replenish sodium and balance electrolytes. My jerky was a big hit during my years as a Boy Scout leader for my sons when they were younger. With a feast of turkey jerky and trail mix, I was a welcomed addition to hikes and campouts.

Wasa (whole grain) crackers with cottage cheese and smoked salmon are a powerhouse of protein, are nutrient dense, and satisfyingly filling. Literally, one full size cracker, a slice of salmon, and a tablespoon of cottage cheese are perfect at about 200 calories. Add a little cracked pepper or a few capers for an extra zip. Substitute tuna salad (made with Veganaise) for the salmon if you prefer.

Avocado is good anytime! Mash a half an avocado (about 150 calories), add a spritz of lemon or lime, and spread on a Wasa cracker or toasted Ezekiel bread squares. Top with a slice of cucumber and cracked pepper. Avocado is excellent in salads and makes a perfect spread for turkey sandwiches. Then there's good old guacamole. Mix avocado with tomatoes, onions, garlic, and lime and you've got one more dip for those veggies we prepped above. There are probably 101 recipes for avocado based snacks. Get creative and make up your own. Let me know what you come up with!

PJ's Favorite Smoothie Recipes

Thanks to all the people who've turned me on to the smoothie revolution!

Some of the recipes below have been adapted from those shared in cookbooks by Jillian Michaels, Gwyneth Paltrow, and Jeff Primack of Qi Revolution. Because of their work in the arena of holistic living, I've come to embrace the whole food movement and smoothie lifestyle. They all had a hand in teaching me the magic and artistry of making delicious, nutritious smoothies. Thanks for spreading the love…

I use a Blendtech mixer for my smoothie recipes and for making nut milks, soups, and nut butters, but a Vitamix will do pretty much the same thing. The Magic Bullet and Ninja blenders will also do the trick for most of these recipes, although for dense veggies like beets, or to make your own almond or coconut milk, high powered blenders with larger reservoirs work best.

Because I'm lactose intolerant and want to use the most nutrient dense ingredients with the least amount of additives, I recently began making my own almond and coconut milk as a base for most of my smoothies. You can get these pre-made non-dairy milks at your local grocer or whole foods store, but check the ingredients to make sure you aren't getting added sugars, carrageenan (a highly inflammatory thickener), or other fillers like "natural flavors." Relatively new to nut milks, I haven't yet tried homemade cashew or hemp milk, but there are recipes for making your own online. Be sure to buy organic raw nuts whenever possible, and avoid genetically modified versions.

I've compiled my smoothie recipes from several sources over the past few years and have modified many of them to suit my own nutritional needs and tastes. I recommend you do the same. Don't be afraid to experiment and add ingredients that blend well and enhance the flavor. Just remember to keep track of the calories since they add up fast when mixing fruits, nut milks, and nut butters. Go for quality rather than quantity to adjust flavors, adding a small amount of natural, nutrient dense, flavorful ingredients.

I'll start with how to make your own homemade nut milks to use as your smoothie base. Almond and coconut milk have a wide range of vitamins and minerals, including iron, selenium, sodium, calcium, magnesium, phosphorous, and potassium. In addition, they are loaded with Vitamins C, E, and B complex. Half the medium chain fatty acids in coconut milk are composed of lauric acid, which is anti-viral, antibacterial, anti-microbial, and antifungal, thus strengthening the immune system. Almond milk is loaded with health benefits as well, including being free of saturated fats and cholesterol. The short and medium chain fatty acids contained in these beverages quickly convert to energy instead of being stored as fat and are even touted with assisting weight loss. Coconut and almond milk are vegan, dairy free, soy free, and gluten free. All good things.

NOTE: I'm not averse to people drinking cow's milk as long as it's free of growth hormones, antibiotics, and that the dairy cows are humanely treated. Organic whole milk is loaded with protein, calcium, vitamin D, and potassium, and has essential vitamins and minerals beneficial for bone growth and necessary for healthy development in children. Alternatives such as goat's milk are also

recommended if children are found to be lactose intolerant. If your child suffers with stomach cramps, constipation, diarrhea, or chronic allergies/ear infections, consider the possibility that he or she is lactose intolerant or lactose sensitive and seek medical advice regarding alternatives.

Homemade Almond Milk

Ingredients:
3 cups filtered water
1 cup almonds (raw/organic is best)

Instructions:

1) Soak almonds overnight in 2 cups of water (not the same water you'll use for blending). Drain and rinse thoroughly the next day. (Almonds can soak for up to two days in the refrigerator).

2) Pour almonds and 3 cups of fresh filtered water into blender. Select "Whole juice" or blend on high speed for 2 minutes or until mixture is smooth and frothy.

3) Pour through a mesh strainer lined with cheesecloth (or purchase a reusable nut milk bag for about $10), and let liquids drain into bowl. Squeeze remaining liquid through cheesecloth or nut milk bag until left with dry almond meal. You have to really squeeze, squeeze, squeeze to get every last drop of goodness, but I find it therapeutic and somehow primal. I actually look forward to going through the process. It only takes about twenty minutes a couple of times per week.

NOTE: You can keep the almond meal if you like and use it later for baking, pie crusts, or put some in your cereal or homemade granola bars. Dry it by spreading it onto a baking pan and baking on low in the oven for up to three hours until it's dry and crumbly. Store in a zip lock bag or plastic container in the freezer for up to six months.

Makes ~4 cups of almond milk. I sometimes double the recipe if I know I'm going to use it up quickly. If you want it thicker, use less water. Use more water for thinner almond milk. If you like it flavored, add a tsp. of vanilla, a TBSP. of agave nectar, or a dash of cinnamon. Store in fridge for up to three days and shake thoroughly before each use. I forego the added agave/sugar. The nutty taste has a natural sweetness that's perfect for me.

Coconut Milk

Ingredients:
4 cups of warm filtered water (or boil and let cool).
1 ½-2 cups of unsweetened shredded coconut (or one raw coconut)

You can buy unsweetened shredded coconut packaged or go through the labor intensive version of draining a real coconut, busting it open with a hammer, soaking the coconut pieces for about 10 minutes to separate it from the outer shell, and then peeling the brown "skin" off the coconut pieces. I, personally, find this a labor of love, but the time investment and risk of injury is certainly greater, and the taste is only marginally better.

Instructions:

1) Heat water, but don't boil. It should be hot, but not scalding.
2) Put coconut meat in blender and add water. (If all water won't fit, you can add the water in two batches. Don't forget to save a half cup or so of water to clean out the blender and get the most of your coconut remnants. Also remember to use the water you drained from the coconut for added flavor and nutrition.)
3) Blend on high for several minutes until thick and creamy.
4) Pour through a mesh colander lined with cheesecloth (or nut milk bag) until liquid has drained through to bowl underneath. Then squeeze through several thicknesses of cheesecloth/mesh bag to get remaining milk out. Squeeze, squeeze, squeeze, until no more liquid comes through. You'll be left with dried coconut in your cheesecloth that doesn't have much flavor. I don't bother saving this.
5) If you have to split the water, pour all the coconut milk that you strained out back into the blender, add the remaining water, and repeat.
6) To flavor (not that it needs it), add ½ tsp vanilla extract, or to make chocolate coconut milk, add 2 tsp cocoa powder + ½ tsp vanilla.
7) Should be used in 3-4 days after making for best flavor and texture. Shake well before using.

Berry Blast Smoothie

Ingredients:
1 cup milk or almond milk
½ cup strawberries (fresh or frozen)
½ cup raspberries (fresh or frozen)
NOTE: I use organic frozen antioxidant berry blend
¼ cup plain Greek yogurt
(1 tsp. honey, agave, or organic maple syrup if you need more sweetness, but really…it doesn't need it)

Instructions:

Add a cup of crushed ice if you're using fresh fruit rather than frozen. Blend on high 1-2 minutes until smooth. For a burst of protein and omega-3s, add 1 tsp. ground flax seed, hemp hearts, or whey protein powder. Makes two servings of about 160 calories each.

Green Choco Monkey Smoothie

Inspired by my addiction to the Coco Monkey Smoothie from the Granby Village Health Food Store in Granby, CT., I've adapted their recipe and added a few twists.

Ingredients:
1 cup Silk Chocolate Almond Milk (or make your own chocolate almond milk by adding 2 tsp. of cocoa powder and a ½ tsp. vanilla extract to your homemade almond milk)

1 TBSP. almond butter (or organic peanut butter)
1 frozen banana (peeled and cut into pieces)
1 scoop Green's Organics Superfood (Amazonian Chocolate) powder. (According to the label, 1 scoop has the nutrients equal to 7 servings of fruits and veggies.)
1 tsp. vanilla extract

Instructions:

Blend all ingredients on high (Smoothie setting on Blendtec) for 45-60 seconds until smooth. Drink and enjoy. Best shake you'll ever taste and packed with nutrition. Makes two servings with about 250 calories each.

Banana Almond Protein Smoothie

This one is a modified version of a Jillian Michaels smoothie recipe from her *Master Your Metabolism Cookbook*. I've added the choice of hemp hearts (love those little suckers for their huge protein content and heart healthy omega-3s). I've also added plant protein and/or maca powder which has a burst of micronutrients and energy boosting vitamins and minerals.

Ingredients:
1 cup unsweetened almond milk
1 small banana
1 TBLSP. almond butter
1 TBLSP. ground flaxseed or hemp hearts
½ scoop plant based protein powder or maca powder
A cup of crushed ice or ice cubes

Instructions:
Blend banana, almond milk, almond butter, flax or hemp, and protein powder on high (Smoothie setting on Blendtec) for 45-60 seconds. Add ice and blend again until smooth. Makes two servings at about 200 calories each.

Tropical Burst Smoothie

Ingredients:
1 cup almond or almond coconut milk
4-5 ripe organic strawberries (fresh or frozen)
1 ripe kiwi (peeled)
½ an orange
½ a lime
Sliced fresh ginger to taste (I like just a hint of ginger so I only use a slice or two)

Instructions:
Blend on high for 45-60seconds. For a thicker smoothie that packs a probiotic punch, add ½ cup of plain kefir.

Also add a sprig of mint to the mix if you want a refreshing burst of an age old digestive soother. Makes two servings of about 150 calories each.

Creamy Avocado & Cocoa Smoothie

This one is straight out of Gwyneth Paltrow's, *It's All Good* cookbook, a staple in any whole foods' kitchen.

Ingredients:
1 ripe avocado, peeled and pitted
1 cup fresh coconut water
1 cup cold, unsweetened almond milk
1 TBLSP. raw cocoa powder
1 heaping TBLSP. ground hemp seeds
1 TBLSP. raw honey (I use Manuka honey or organic maple syrup)

Instructions:

Blend all ingredients together on high for 45-60 seconds until smooth or choose "Whole juice" on your Blendtec. Drink immediately. Makes two servings of about 300 calories each.

Thanks Gwyneth! I love this one. Look for more of Ms. Paltrow's smoothie recipes in her cook book.

Beets & Greens Smoothie

This one is my own concoction and has taken some time to perfect. Greens like kale and spinach have tons of necessary vitamins and minerals. There's far more calcium in our leafy pals than there is in dairy and none of the inflammatory properties. They are loaded with phytonutrients that have many healing benefits to the body and should be eaten often. Since our American diets don't consist of nearly enough of these green leafy superfoods, juicing and adding them to smoothies is a great way to fit them in. However, greens can have a very…um…earthy taste. Beets and root vegetables, too, are loaded with micronutrients, minerals, and antioxidants. But adding even a slice of beet to your smoothie or juice can make it downright unpalatable. I've discovered some tricks to getting these all important veggies into my diet.

Ingredients:

8 ounces filtered water
½ a small fresh beet (cut in two pieces) **NOTE: A little bit of beet goes a long way for flavor. It's also a potent liver cleanser so more is not better.**
1 cup of kale leaves chopped (I prefer to use baby kale and remove the center stems or ribs)
1 large carrot (cut into pieces)
1 large apple (cut into wedges)
½ avocado (peeled and pitted)
A slice of lemon (peel and pith removed)

A 1 inch slice of fresh ginger root
½ cup ice (tastes best when cold)

Instructions:

Blend all ingredients on high for 1-2 minutes or until smooth, or use the "Whole juice" setting on your Blendtec. The result is a thick, creamy, smoothie with a bit of a bite and a gently sweet aftertaste. I drink it as a meal replacement on days when I'm on the road through lunch and don't want to be tempted to eat out. It's filling, nutritious, and dare I say…tasty.

I love hearing about new smoothie recipes so if you have one to share, visit my website and leave me a note on [my contact page](), or find me on [Facebook]() or [twitter]() and spread the smoothie love!

Final Note

So there you have it. My best tips, tricks, and ideas for staying healthy and happy while you're writing, reading, or otherwise sitting your way to fulfilling your dreams. I understand that change isn't easy, but I encourage you to define what is most important to you in life and then make a plan to become the best you that you can be, so that whatever your dreams are, you'll have the tools you need to achieve them. Start small, stick with it, and keep learning new ways to help you and your loved ones overcome a sedentary lifestyle.

Hopefully, I've given you enough simple tools that you can easily incorporate them into your life without too much angst. Apply what works for you and adopt the "easy stuff" first. Set yourself up for success by setting clear, manageable, measurable goals and finding supporters who will hold you accountable. We aren't alone in this fight and there truly is strength in numbers. Getting healthy and staying healthy doesn't have to be a painful process. Try to have fun with it and avoid adding the pressure of trying to be "perfect."

None of us does it "right" all the time and we shouldn't expect perfection from ourselves or anyone else, but with each positive choice you make, you are one step closer to living the life you want to live. I often tell my clients to treat themselves the way they would treat a best friend. Be kind, generous, and loving toward yourself and others, and you will be rewarded with a sense of peace and happiness that only comes from spreading love from the deepest part of your soul. Open your heart and mind, and be willing to change at your very core. This willingness to change and grow is at the heart of evolving into the person you were truly meant to be.

Believing you deserve a happy, healthy, prosperous life is the first step to attaining it.

Stand up for your life!

I hope you've found this book helpful and that you'll recommend it to friends and family. Word of mouth and positive reviews are the best way to thank authors for creating great books. I'd greatly appreciate it if you could take a moment and leave a review on Goodreads and Amazon.

Thank you, and may you be blessed with peace and abundance in all you do.

ABOUT THE AUTHOR

More about PJ

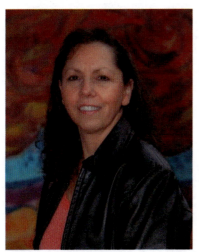

In addition to authoring award winning young adult novels, PJ Sharon owns ABSolute Fitness and Therapeutic Bodywork, a private practice massage therapy and personal training business in East Granby, CT. With over twenty-five years in the health and fitness industry, Ms. Sharon offers a multidisciplinary approach to wellness.

As a Physical Therapist Assistant (PTA), Massage Therapist (LMT), Certified Personal Fitness Trainer (CPFT), and Yoga Instructor, Ms. Sharon brings a wealth of knowledge to her clients and workshops. A graduate of Springfield Technical Community College and the Connecticut Center for Massage Therapy, Ms. Sharon also holds certifications as a trainer through the NFPT and teaches therapeutic yoga. A Black Belt in the art of Shaolin Kempo Karate and former figure skating and power skating instructor, Ms. Sharon's passion for holistic health and healing comes through in her writing—whether she is penning romantic and hopeful stories for teens or sharing her wisdom and experience with clients and workshop attendees.

When she's not writing or spreading the love through her practice, she can be found kayaking in the Berkshire Hills of Massachusetts and renovating an old farmhouse with the love of her life.

Author contact info and social media sites:

Website: http://www.pjsharon.com

Follow PJ on Twitter: @pjsharon   http://www.twitter.com/pjsharon

"Like" PJ on Facebook: http://www.facebook.com/pjsharonbooks

Signup for PJ's Newsletter at her website: http://eepurl.com/bm7rj5

Other books by PJ Sharon

Aside from writing and publishing her debut non-fiction book, OVERCOME your SEDENTARY LIFESTYLE (A Practical Guide to Improving Health, Fitness, and Well-being for Desk Dwellers and Couch Potatoes), PJ Sharon is an award winning author of young adult books, including PIECES of LOVE, HEAVEN is for HEROES, ON THIN ICE, and Holt Medallion winner SAVAGE CINDERELLA. Ms. Sharon loves writing for teens and teens at heart. Her latest work, HEALING WATERS, completes The Chronicles of Lily Carmichael, a YA dystopian trilogy that RT Book Reviews calls ***"An action-packed read with a strong female lead."*** Ms. Sharon is a *Library Journal's* Self-e selected author. For more info on PJ's books and updates on new releases, sign up for her newsletter or visit her website.

Signup for PJ's Newsletter: http://eepurl.com/bm7rj5

Visit PJ's Website for more information and buy links: http://www.pjsharon.com

Young Adult Fiction Titles

NOVELS

Contemporary Young Adult:

Pieces of Love, Heaven is for Heroes, On Thin Ice, and Savage Cinderella

Dystopian (Sci-fi/fantasy) Young Adult:

Chronicles of Lily Carmichael trilogy

Book One—Waning Moon

Book Two—Western Desert

Book Three—Healing Waters

SHORTS

Soul Redemption—15k Short story prequel to WANING MOON

Sami's Christmas Wish List—28k novella (Girls of Thompson Lake Box Set available in e-book only)

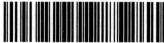

Made in the USA
Charleston, SC
02 January 2016